Pediatric Transfusion: A Physician's Handbook

First Edition

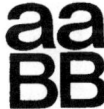

American Association of Blood Banks
2003

To purchase additional copies of this book, please call our sales department at (301)215-6499 or fax orders to (301)907-6895. AABB sales representatives are available from 8:30 am to 5:00 pm ET, Monday through Friday, for telephone access. For other book services, including chapter reprints and large quantity sales, ask for the Senior Sales Associate. Visit the American Association of Blood Banks Web site on the Internet at www.aabb.org or email our sales department at sales@aabb.org.

Mention of specific products or equipment by contributors to this AABB publication does not represent an endorsement of such products by the AABB nor does it necessarily indicate a preference for those products over other similar competitive products. Any forms and/or procedures in this book are examples. AABB does not imply or guarantee that the materials meet federal, state, or other applicable requirements. It is incumbent on the reader who intends to use any information, forms, policies, or procedures contained in this publication to evaluate such materials for use in light of particular circumstances associated with their institution.

Efforts are made to have publications of the AABB consistent in regard to acceptable practices. However, for several reasons, they may not be. First, as new developments in the practice of blood banking occur, changes may be recommended to the *Standards for Blood Banks and Transfusion Services*. It is not possible, however, to revise each publication at the time such a change is adopted. Thus, it is essential that the most recent edition of the *Standards* be consulted as a reference in regard to current acceptable practices. Second, the views expressed in this publication represent the opinions of authors. The publication of this book does not constitute an endorsement by the AABB of any view expressed herein, and the AABB expressly disclaims any liability arising from any inaccuracy or misstatement.

Editor

Susan D. Roseff, MD

Contributing Editors

Linda Chambers, MD
Anne Eder, MD, PhD
Patricia Pisciotto, MD
Steven Sloan, MD, PhD
Ronald Strauss, MD

Handbook Series Editor

Darrell J. Triulzi, MD

Copyright © 2003
American Association of Blood Banks

All rights reserved. No part of this book may be reproduced or transmitted in any form or by any means, electronic or mechanical, including photocopying, recording, or by any information storage and retrieval systems, without permission in writing from:

American Association of Blood Banks
8101 Glenbrook Road
Bethesda, Maryland 20814

ISBN NO. 1-56395-180-0
Printed in the United States of America
2003

Contents

Preface vii

BLOOD COMPONENTS 1

Concept of Component Therapy 1
Red Blood Cells 1
Red Blood Cells Washed 16
Platelets 17
Plasma Components 23
Cryoprecipitated Antihemophilic Factor 29
Granulocytes 31
Whole Blood 36
Donor-Specific Units 36
Component Therapy for Patients Undergoing
  Extracorporeal Membrane Oxygenation 39
References 40

ALLOIMMUNE CYTOPENIAS 51

Overview of Alloimmune Cytopenias 51
Immune-Mediated Hemolytic Disease
  of the Fetus and Newborn 51
Neonatal Alloimmune Thrombocytopenia 66
Neonatal Alloimmune Neutropenia 70
Alloimmune Cytopenias Resulting from Blood
  Transfusion Therapy 72
Transfusion Support Following ABO-Incompatible
  Hematopoietic Transplantation 81
References 84

HEMOSTATIC DISORDERS 91

Overview of Hemostasis 91
Platelet Function 91
Factor VIII Preparations for von Willebrand
  Disease 93
The Procoagulant System 94
The Procoagulant System in Neonates 95

Abnormalities of the Procoagulant System 98
The Anticoagulant and Fibrinolytic Systems 105
References 108

ADVERSE EFFECTS OF BLOOD TRANSFUSION 113

Acute Transfusion Reactions 113
Delayed Transfusion Reactions 136
References 143

SPECIAL PRODUCTS 149

Overview of Special Products 149
CMV-Reduced-Risk Components 149
Gamma-Irradiated Components 153
Leukocyte-Reduced Components 157
Components that Are Negative for Sickle
    Hemoglobin 159
References 161

Index 165

Preface

On a regular basis, the American Association of Blood Banks (AABB) receives inquiries from neonatologists and pediatricians who would like a concise yet comprehensive resource to guide their transfusion practices. In addition, many specialists within the field of transfusion medicine are daunted by questions relating to the special considerations in transfusing infants and small children. This book has been designed to fill the needs of all practitioners who transfuse the neonatal and pediatric populations.

Pediatric Transfusion: A Physician's Handbook is intended to serve as a resource for physicians treating patients in the hospital or those answering questions while on call in the blood bank. The contributors have a wealth of practical experience to share, and they have included as much detail as possible—especially with regard to volumes of blood components and doses of medication for these tiny patients.

The book has been written in the handbook format so it can be carried conveniently in a lab coat pocket. In order to keep the text concise, some background material has been omitted. *Blood Transfusion Therapy: A Physician's Handbook* can be used as a companion, to fill in some of the details of basic transfusion medicine that are applicable to both adult and pediatric patients. For the detail that a handbook cannot encompass, readers are referred to the AABB *Technical Manual* and *Pediatric Transfusion Therapy* (AABB Press), as well as the referenced publications at the end of each chapter.

The hard work of all the contributing editors is deeply appreciated, on this, our first edition. Special thanks go to Janet McGrath and other members of the AABB staff who supported us through the project. Comments from readers are encouraged so future editions can be further tailored to meet everyone's needs.

BLOOD COMPONENTS

Concept of Component Therapy

Hospitalized preterm infants represent one of the most frequently transfused populations in tertiary care hospitals. This chapter discusses component therapy for patients less than 18 years old. Special consideration is given to neonates who are less than 4 months old. A "preterm" infant is any neonate whose birth occurs through the end of the last day of the 37th week (259th day) following the onset of the last menstrual period of the mother.[1]

Most blood is separated into components before transfusion.[2] These components are listed in Table 1.[2-5] Separation of blood into components offers several advantages. First, this procedure conserves blood resources because one donated unit can benefit several patients. Second, separation of whole blood into components allows for optimal storage conditions of each component. Third, transfusion of blood components provides the optimal method of transfusing patients who require large amounts of a specific component.

Red Blood Cells

Description of Component

One Red Blood Cell (RBC) unit is about 300 mL containing approximately 200 mL of erythrocytes, approximately 50 mL of plasma, and an anticoagulant-preservative solution.[2] Several anti-

Table 1. Blood Components and Plasma Derivatives*

Component/Product (Volume)	Composition	Usual Indications
Red Blood Cells in CPD, CP2D, CPDA-1 (~250 mL)	RBCs (approx. Hct 75%); 50-70 mL plasma, WBCs, and platelets (dysfunctional)	Increase red cell mass in symptomatic anemia
Red Blood Cells with additive solution (~330 mL)	RBCs (approx. Hct 60%); 40 mL plasma, WBCs, and platelets (dysfunctional); 100 mL of additive solution	Increase red cell mass in symptomatic anemia
Red Blood Cells Leukocytes Reduced (~300 mL with additive) (~225 mL without additive)	Approx. Hct 60% (additive unit); Hct 75% (without additive); $<5 \times 10^6$ WBCs; few dysfunctional platelets; 40 mL plasma	Increase red cell mass; $<5 \times 10^6$ WBCs decreases the likelihood of febrile reactions, immunization to leukocytes (HLA antigens), or CMV transmission
Red Blood Cells Washed (~180 mL)	RBCs (approx. Hct 75%); $<5 \times 10^8$ WBCs; no plasma	Increase red cell mass; reduce risk of allergic reactions to plasma proteins, reduced potassium, decreased additives
Granulocytes Pheresis (~220 mL)	Granulocytes ($>1.0 \times 10^{10}$ PMN/unit); lymphocytes; platelets ($>2.0 \times 10^{11}$/unit); some RBCs. 3 to 8 times greater granulocyte content from stimulated donors[3,4]	Provide granulocytes for selected patients with sepsis and severe neutropenia (<500 PMN/μL)

Platelets (~50 mL)	Platelets (>5.5 × 10^{10}/unit); ~50 mL plasma; RBCs; WBCs	Bleeding caused by thrombocytopenia or thrombocytopathy
Platelets Pheresis (~300 mL)	Platelets (>3 × 10^{11}/unit); ~300 mL plasma; RBCs; WBCs	Same as Platelets; sometimes HLA matched or crossmatch compatible
Platelets Leukocytes Reduced (~300 mL)	Platelets (as above); <5 × 10^6 WBCs	Same as Platelets; <5 × 10^6 WBCs to decrease the likelihood of febrile reactions, alloimmunization to leukocytes (HLA antigens), or CMV transmission
FFP (~220 mL)	Plasma; all coagulation factors; complement (no platelets)	Treatment of some coagulation disorders
Cryoprecipitated AHF (~15 mL)	Fibrinogen; ≥ 150 mg Factor VIII; ≥ 80 IU Factor XIII von Willebrand factor	Deficiency or dysfunction of fibrinogen or Factor XIII; von Willebrand disease (in the absence of a safer alternative)
Albumin 20 mL, 50 mL, 250 mL sizes available	Albumin (5% or 25%), some α-, β-globulins	Volume expansion

(continued)

Table 1. Blood Components and Plasma Derivatives* (continued)

Component/Product (Volume)	Composition	Usual Indications
Rh Immune Globulin Various doses from 50 to 1000 μg in volumes from 1 to 8.5 mL	IgG anti-D; preparations for IV or IM use or both	Prevention of D antibody formation; 18 μg IV/mL of RBC exposure or 20 to 24 μg IM/mL of RBC exposure depending on specific product Treatment of autoimmune thrombocytopenia; 25 to 50 μg/kg IV is the recommended initial dose
Whole Blood (500 mL)	RBCs (approx. Hct 40%); 200 mL plasma; (deficient in labile clotting Factors V and VIII); platelets (dysfunctional); WBCs	Increase both red cell mass and plasma volume

*Table is adapted from Triulzi, ed.[5]

RBCs = red blood cells; Hct = hematocrit; WBCs = white blood cells; CMV = cytomegalovirus; PMN = polymorphonuclear cells; FFP = fresh frozen plasma; IV = intravenous; IM = intramuscular; AHF = antihemophilic factor.

coagulant-preservative solutions are used in the United States, with most incorporating additive solutions for extended preservation of red cells. The additive solutions contain dextrose, adenine, sodium chloride (and sometimes sodium phosphate), mannitol, sodium citrate, and citric acid. The hematocrit of an RBC unit is 52% to 60%. If the collection system does not include an additive solution, the hematocrit of an RBC unit is 70% to 80%. RBCs are not a source of functional platelets or granulocytes and provide only small amounts of clotting factors and other plasma proteins.

Indications

RBCs are indicated for treatment of anemia in patients who require an increase in oxygen-carrying capacity. The transfusion requirements of each patient should be based on the patient's hemoglobin and hematocrit levels, symptoms of anemia, and risk factors (Table 2).

For most children, RBC transfusions should be considered after an acute blood loss of approximately 15% to 20% of their blood volume.[6,7] With acute blood losses, such as those that occur in trauma or during surgery, the hemoglobin and hematocrit may not reflect the extent of blood loss. Rather, evidence of hypoperfusion, such as pallor, hypotension, tachycardia, and decreased mental status, should be used to determine the appropriate replacement therapy. Patients with chronic anemia often can tolerate relatively severe anemia because their bodies compensate without the need for transfusion. A child older than 1 year with a healthy cardiovascular system will be able to tolerate hemoglobin levels of 7 to 8 g/dL. Neonates and patients with sickle cell anemia or thalassemia deserve special consideration (see Alloimmune Cytopenias).

Neonates

In the first few days of life, full-term neonates normally have an elevated hemoglobin level of 14 to 20 g/dL. Those born after delayed cord clamping tend to have even higher levels.[8] Over the first 2 to 3 months of life, the hemoglobin levels normally decrease to a

Table 2. Guidelines for Transfusion of RBCs in Patients More than 4 Months of Age*

1. Intraoperative blood loss ≥15% total blood volume (TBV)
2. Hemoglobin <8 g/dL
   - In perioperative period, with symptoms of anemia
   - In chemotherapy or radiotherapy
   - In chronic congenital or acquired symptomatic anemia
   - In emergency surgical procedures with expected blood loss in patient with significant preoperative anemia
   - In preoperative anemia when other corrective therapy is not available
3. Acute blood loss with hypovolemia not responsive to other therapy
4. Hemoglobin <13 g/dL with
   - Severe pulmonary disease
   - ECMO
5. Chronic transfusion programs for disorders of red cell production (such as β-thalassemia major and Diamond-Blackfan syndrome unresponsive to therapy)

*Adapted with permission from Roseff, Luban, Manno.[6]

nadir of about 11 to 12 g/dL and then gradually rise.[8] Even with near-normal levels of erythrocytes, the hemoglobin of neonates is predominantly hemoglobin F, which is relatively poor at delivering oxygen to tissues. Hence, some neonates may benefit from transfusion of RBCs despite the fact that they are not very anemic. As with all patients, the decision to transfuse RBCs should be based on the neonate's clinical situation. Symptoms associated with anemia in neonates may include tachypnea, tachycardia, dyspnea, apnea episodes, and periods of diminished activity. The guidelines outlined in Table 3 summarize expert opinions that are based on the limited studies published in this area. Neonates with

Table 3. Guidelines for Transfusion of RBCs in Patients Less than 4 Months of Age*

1. Hemoglobin <7 g/dL with low reticulocyte count and symptoms of anemia[†]
2. Hemoglobin <10 g/dL with an infant
   - On <35% hood O_2
   - On O_2 by nasal cannula
   - On continuous positive airway pressure (CPAP)/intermittent mandatory ventilation (IMV) with mechanical ventilation with mean airway pressure <6 cm H_2O
   - Significant apnea or bradycardia[‡]
   - Significant tachycardia or tachypnea[§]
   - Low weight gain[‖]
3. Hemoglobin <12 g/dL with an infant
   - On >35% hood O_2
   - On CPAP/IMV with mean airway pressure ≥6 to 8 cm H_2O
4. Hemoglobin <15 g/dL with an infant
   - On extracorporeal membrane oxygenation (ECMO)
   - Congenital cyanotic heart disease

*Adapted from Roseff, Luban, Manno.[6]
[†]Tachycardia, tachypnea, poor feeding.
[‡]>6 episodes in 12 hours or 2 episodes in 24 hours requiring bag and mask ventilation while receiving therapeutic doses of methylxanthines.
[§]Heart rate >180 beats/minute for 24 hours; respiratory rate >80 breaths/minute for 24 hours.
[‖]Gain of <10 g/day observed over 4 days while receiving ≥100 kcal/kg/day.

severe pulmonary or cardiac disease may benefit from transfusions aimed at maintaining a hemoglobin level of 13 g/dL.[9,10]

Premature Infants

Premature infants are born with an anemia proportional to their degree of prematurity. Infants with birthweights of 1.0 to 1.5 kg have a mean hemoglobin concentration of about 8 g/dL, whereas infants with birthweights less than 1 kg have a mean hemoglobin concentration of 7 g/dL.[11,12] As is the case with full-term infants, the hemoglobin concentrations of premature infants decrease during the first few months of life. However, in comparison to full-term infants, premature infants develop a more profound decrease in hemoglobin concentration as a result of frequent blood sampling, management of medical complications, and a diminished capacity to increase plasma erythropoietin.[13] Because of their diminished capacity to make erythropoietin, premature infants are more likely to have low reticulocyte counts and may benefit from transfusions at hemoglobin concentrations of approximately 7 g/dL (Table 3).

Congenital Hemoglobinopathies

Patients with congenital hemoglobinopathies are unusual because of their need, often from childhood, for chronic transfusion.

Sickle Cell Disease. Because of the high likelihood of the development of alloimmunization to red cell antigens in patients who have sickle cell disease and who require regular transfusion, specific transfusion requirements are discussed in Alloimmune Cytopenias.

Thalassemia. Patients with thalassemia major require transfusion support to manage their disease. In these patients, the goal of RBC transfusions is not only to provide oxygen-carrying capacity but also to suppress endogenous erythropoiesis that causes bony abnormalities. To accomplish this goal, most patients are transfused every 3 to 4 weeks at a dose that maintains a pretransfusion hemoglobin concentration of 9.5 to 10.5 g/dL and a posttransfusion hemoglobin concentration of 13 to 13.5 g/dL.[14] Chronic transfusion therapy causes toxic iron overload, and there have been some attempts to reduce the number of transfusions by transfusing young red cells that have a longer lifespan. However, large studies have failed to show any benefit of this approach, and it is not recommended.[15]

Selection of RBCs—Immunologic Considerations

Patients Older than 4 Months

Transfused RBCs must be ABO compatible with the patient (Table 4). Although all patients can receive group O RBCs, most patients receive group-specific RBC units. D-positive patients can receive D-negative or D-positive RBCs. However, D-negative patients should receive D-negative RBCs to prevent an immune response to the D antigen. Such an immune response may result in delayed extravascular hemolysis and may complicate future transfusions or pregnancies.[2,5]

In addition to compatibility with ABO and D antigens, patients can make antibodies to a large variety of other antigens on the surface of erythrocytes. Clinically important antibodies that can cause hemolysis are stimulated by exposure to foreign antigens during transfusion, pregnancy, or organ or marrow trans-

Table 4. ABO Selection of Blood Components

Patient ABO Type	Antibody (Serum)	RBCs or Granulocytes	Plasma-Containing Components*	Whole Blood
O (45%)	Anti-A and Anti-B	O	A, B, AB, O	O
A (40%)	Anti-B	A, O	A, AB	A
B (11%)	Anti-A	B, O	B, AB	B
AB (4%)	None	A, B, AB, O	AB	AB

*For neonates and patients undergoing human progenitor cell transplantation, it is preferable to transfuse platelets containing plasma that is ABO compatible with the recipient.

plantation. To prevent hemolysis from such unexpected antibodies, an antibody screen of each patient's serum is conducted. Clinically significant antibodies are identified, and units lacking the corresponding antigens are selected for transfusion. Finally, the selected units are crossmatched to ensure that each RBC unit is compatible with the patient.[2,5]

Neonates

Special considerations apply when selecting RBC units for neonates.

ABO Groups. Neonatal blood contains maternal immunoglobulins in its serum, some of which may be directed against the A, B, or both antigens, depending on the maternal blood group. In addition to being compatible with the infant's blood group, the transfused red cells must be compatible with the maternal blood group. For simplicity, many transfusion services transfuse group O RBCs to all neonates. To conserve group O RBC units, which serve as "universal donor" units used in emergencies, some blood banks dispense type-specific blood if sensitive tests demonstrate that the neonate's serum lacks maternal antibodies directed against neonatal blood group antigens.[2]

Antibody Screen. The antibody screen for unexpected antibodies must be performed before selecting RBC units for neonatal transfusion. Because the antibodies in neonatal blood are of maternal origin, maternal blood often serves as the source of serum for the antibody screen, although neonatal blood can be used. Furthermore, because the neonatal immune system rarely produces antibodies in response to RBC transfusions, antibody screens need not be repeated during the hospitalization of a neonate.[2]

Dosage and Rate of Administration. A transfusion of 10 to 15 mL/kg of RBCs will raise the hemoglobin concentration by about 2 to 3 g/dL (Table 5). The transfusion usually is administered over 1 to 2 hours but must be completed within 4 hours. The rate can be adjusted according to the patient's clinical status and needs.[2,6]

Table 5. Standard Transfusion Volumes for Children*

Component	Volume	Estimated Change
RBCs	10 to 15 mL/kg	Hb ↑ 2 to 3 g/dL
Platelets	5 to 10 mL/kg	Platelets ↑ 50,000 to 100,000/µL
Granulocytes	$\geq 1 \times 10^9$ neutrophils/kg in volume of 15 mL/kg	Repeat until clinical response
FFP	10 to 15 mL/kg	Factor activity ↑ 15% to 20%
Cryoprecipitated AHF	1 to 2 units/10 kg	Fibrinogen ↑ 60 to 100 mg/dL

*Modified with permission from Brecher.[2]

The AABB *Standards for Blood Banks and Transfusion Services* (*Standards*) requires that there is a filter between the blood recipient and any transfused products.[16] For RBC transfusions, 170- to 260-micron filters are included in blood administration sets. A 20- to 40-micron microaggregate filter may be used to remove degenerating platelets, leukocytes, and fibrin strands, but these filters are not in common use. Bedside filtration is not always possible because of the logistics of small-volume transfusions required for some infants and young children and variations in the system used in particular institutions. Most transfusion services chose to consider the filtration done in the transfusion service, at the time of dispensing, as the final filtration step. Concern about whether this practice was in compliance with AABB *Standards* was clarified in the final edition of the *Accreditation Requirements Manual* of the AABB. This publication states that only one filtration step is necessary for infant transfusion; this step may occur either between the syringe and the infant or between the blood container and the syringe, immediately before dispensing the aliquot.[17] If the filtration occurs in an open system, the unit must be transfused within 4 hours.[2]

Special Considerations and Modification of RBCs

Infants

Blood Additives. Additive solutions are used for the preservation and storage of most RBC units. Additive solutions provide both nutrients and a buffer that will preserve the red cells and extend the allowable shelf life to 42 days. The concentrations of the constituents of additive solutions licensed for use in the United States are shown in Table 6.[18] The concentrations of additives present in RBC units are safe for most children and for neonates receiving simple transfusions of up to 20 mL/kg.[19] The safety of these solutions has not been proven for extremely ill premature infants with renal or hepatic insufficiency or both or for massive transfusion of neonates during exchange transfusions, extracorporeal membrane oxygenation (ECMO), and cardiopulmonary bypass.[20] There have been concerns about the concentrations of adenine and mannitol, which can cause nephrotoxicity in laboratory animals when used in high concentrations, as well as about the diuretic effects of mannitol and its possible effects on intracerebral pressure. Some institutions provide nonadditive units (CPD, CPDA-1, or C2PD) in these circumstances, but these institutions may require a special order because most RBCs are stored in additive solutions. However, this effort may be unnecessary in light of growing anecdotal reports of the use of additive solutions in large-volume transfusion without adverse effects.[21,22]

Dedicated Units for Serial Neonatal Transfusions. Some premature infants develop anemia and require multiple transfusions of 5 to 20 mL/kg for several weeks. Some transfusion services reserve a fresh unit of RBCs for these patients early in their hospitalization and dispense an aliquot of that unit for each transfusion. Many hospitals that perform this service will reserve one unit for more than one neonate to conserve resources. Some concerns have been voiced about these programs. Preparation of aliquots requires the use of sterile connecting devices and many blood banks do not own such devices. Additionally, a patho-

Table 6. Formulation of Anticoagulant-Preservative Solutions in Blood Collection Sets[18]

Constituent	CPDA	AS-1	AS-3	AS-5
Volume (mL)	63*	100†	100†	100†
Sodium chloride (mg)	None	900	410	877
Dextrose (mg)	2000	2200	1100	900
Adenine (mg)	17.3	27	30	30
Mannitol (mg)	None	750	None	525
Trisodium citrate (mg)	1660	None	588	None
Citric acid (mg)	206	None	42	None
Sodium phosphate (monobasic) (mg)	140	None	276	None

*Approximately 450 mL of donor blood is drawn into 63 mL of CPDA. A unit of RBCs (hematocrit of about 70%) is prepared by centrifugation and removal of most plasma.
†When AS-1 or AS-5 is used, 450 mL of donor blood is first drawn into 63 mL of CPD, which is identical to CPDA, except that it contains 1610 mg of dextrose per 63 mL and has no adenine. When AS-3 is used, donor blood is drawn into CP2D, which is identical to CPD, except it contains double the amount of dextrose. After centrifugation and removal of nearly all plasma, RBCs are resuspended in 100 mL of the additive solution (AS-1, AS-3, or AS-5) at a hematocrit of 55% to 60%.

gen-contaminated unit could infect more patients because it would be transfused to more than one patient. A final concern is that if a reserved RBC unit is contaminated, the patient may receive several doses of that pathogen. Despite these concerns, those blood banks that have invested in such a program have found that it can be an effective method of minimizing donor exposures and have not detected increased adverse events associated with directed units for serial neonatal transfusion. In addition, these programs have been found to be cost effective.[23-25]

Age of RBCs. During storage of RBCs, erythrocytes leak potassium and consume 2,3-diphosphoglycerate (2,3-DPG) (see

Table 7 and Adverse Effects of Blood Transfusion).[2] Although these changes are not a consideration for most patients, high extracellular potassium loads may be a concern for infants and especially neonates receiving massive transfusions, such as those that occur during ECMO, cardiopulmonary bypass, or exchange transfusion. Thus, some transfusion services provide RBC units that are less than 7 to 14 days old for neonates undergoing such procedures. ECMO is discussed further at the end of this chapter.

All Patients

Leukocyte Reduction. Units of RBCs contain 1 to 3×10^9 leukocytes.[26,27] The AABB *Standards* specifies that leukocyte-reduced RBCs contain less than 5×10^6 leukocytes/unit while retaining 85% of the original red cells.[16] The standard 170-micron blood filter does not remove leukocytes, and a special leukocyte reduction filter is required. Leukocyte reduction by filtration may be performed shortly after collection (prestorage filtration), in the trans-

Table 7. RBC Storage Changes*

		Expiration	
Time Point	**Collection**	**Nonadditive†** (35 days)	**Additive‡** (42 days)
pH (measured at 37 C)	7.55	6.71	6.60
2,3-DPG (% of initial value)	100.00	<10.00	<5.00
Plasma K+ (mmol/L)	5.10	78.50‡	50.00

*Used with permission from Brecher.[2]
†Nonadditive units are CPDA-1 units and additive units are AS-1 units. Values are similar for units containing other additive solutions.
‡Value for plasma potassium concentration may appear high in 35-day stored RBC units; the total plasma in these units is only about 70 mL.

fusion service before issue (laboratory filtration), or at the time of transfusion (bedside transfusion). Bedside leukocyte reduction can be inconsistent because of the lack of quality control and lack of standardized procedures. The main disadvantage of poststorage filtration is that leukocytes can release cytokines during storage. Prestorage leukocyte reduction does not have this drawback and may be associated with a lower incidence of febrile transfusion reactions.[28,29]

Leukocyte reduction has three proven benefits and one possible benefit. Leukocyte reduction reduces transmission of cytomegalovirus (see Special Products), reduces alloimmunization to HLA antigens (see Alloimmune Cytopenias), and reduces the incidence of febrile transfusion reactions (see Adverse Effects of Blood Transfusion). Leukocyte reduction also may prevent immunomodulation induced by transfusions.[30] However, posttransfusion immunomodulation has been only partially studied in children; thus, this is not a universally accepted indication in the pediatric population.[31,32]

Some blood suppliers and transfusion services provide exclusively leukocyte-reduced RBCs and platelets. The only medical disadvantage to leukocyte reduction is the loss of 5% to 10% of the red cells from the transfused unit. In addition, this process adds expense that may not be medically justified for all patients.[2,5]

Irradiation. RBCs (and all blood components) must be gamma irradiated with a minimum of 25 Gy when it is necessary to prevent transfusion-associated graft-vs-host disease (see Adverse Effects of Blood Transfusion and Special Products). Irradiated RBCs have a shelf life that is reduced to no more than 28 days following irradiation. The rate of potassium leakage from erythrocytes is increased during the first few days following irradiation. Compared with a nonirradiated RBC unit, the concentration of potassium in the supernatant of an additive unit is about 10 mM higher 2 days following irradiation and 20 mM higher after about 5 days of storage.[33-35] To estimate the total extracellular potassium transfused to a patient, one must know that a unit of RBCs stored in additive solutions contains approximately 130 mL of supernatant. Compared with additive RBC units, non-additive units contain about the same total amount of potassium in the supernatant, but the potassium concentration is higher in nonadditive units because they contain less supernatant. For infants, the volume of an aliquot must be taken into account.

Red Blood Cells Washed

Description of Component

RBCs may be washed and resuspended with sterile saline, usually at hematocrits of 70% to 80% with a volume of approximately 220 mL. A standard washing procedure using saline removes about 98% of the plasma. Saline washing usually is performed near the time of transfusion of the component. If washing is performed in an open system, the resultant red cell component can be stored for only 24 hours at 1 to 6 C.

Indications

Washing should not be done routinely and is indicated only in unusual circumstances.[2] Washed RBCs should be considered for an infant who is receiving a rapid infusion of a large-volume transfusion (>20 mL/kg) of older RBCs, because of the risk of hyperkalemia-induced cardiac arrhythmias. Small or premature infants who have recently had cardiac surgery and have intracardiac or central venous catheters or both are at greatest risk. For these patients, many blood banks use blood less than 5 to 14 days old and reserve washing for older products. However, RBCs should be transfused soon after washing because electrolytes can leak rapidly from erythrocytes after washing.

Washing is also recommended to remove plasma proteins in blood components for patients who experience recurrent and severe allergic transfusion reactions.[2,5] This washing includes some patients with IgA deficiency who can develop anaphylaxis (see Adverse Effects of Blood Transfusion). Additives can also be removed by washing if there are safety concerns, although this is probably unnecessary.

Other Treatments for Anemia

Anemia caused by iron or folate deficiency should be treated by dietary supplementation. In some patients, erythropoietin can be used to stimulate erythropoiesis and to reduce the number of transfusions. This step is particularly useful in children with renal disease,[36] those undergoing treatment for solid or hematologic tumors, or those recovering from hematopoietic progenitor cell transplantation.[37-40] The dose of erythropoietin needs to be titrated for each patient, with starting doses of 50 U/kg, subcutaneously, three times per week suggested for most children.[41] Erythropoietin also stimulates erythropoiesis in premature infants, but it is metabolized faster and has an increased plasma volume of distribution. For this reason, it must be administered at higher doses of approximately 200 to 400 U/kg three times per week. At this dose range, erythropoietin enhances hematopoiesis in premature infants. However, the number of transfusions is only marginally decreased and premature infants still require multiple transfusions.[42-45] One adverse effect that has been reported with erythropoietin therapy is pure red-cell aplasia secondary to erythropoietin antibody formation.[46,47]

Platelets

Description of Component

Platelets can be prepared in two different processes. Platelets (PLTs) is the name used for the component prepared by centrifugation of whole blood after its collection. Platelets Pheresis (PP) is the product obtained when donor blood is processed by automated apheresis equipment, which extracts the desired component and returns the remainder of the blood to the donor. When prepared from a whole blood donation by centrifugation, each unit of PLTs must contain at least 5.5×10^{10} platelets, although typical yields are 7 to 9×10^{10}. For larger children and adults, between 3 and 6 units of PLTs are pooled together to constitute one "dose" of platelets.[2,5,16] PLTs are suitable for infants and small children because of the small volume of the component, about 50 to 70 mL.[48]

PP components collected by automated apheresis must contain at least 3×10^{11} platelets, although again, this figure represents a minimum, with higher yields obtained by some blood collection facilities.[2,5,16] One donation represents at least one "dose" of platelets for a large child or average adult and is comparable to 3 to 6 units of whole-blood-derived platelets. PP units are also referred to as "apheresis platelets" or "single-donor platelets." Because one dose of platelets is collected from one donor, PP units confer less infectious exposure than PLTs. The volume of a unit of PP is about 200 mL, larger than is necessary for small children and infants.[48] When HLA-matched, crossmatch-compatible, or antigen-negative platelets are required, they are collected by apheresis.[2,5]

Both types of platelet preparations have a shelf life of 5 days and are stored at room temperature (20 to 24 C). They must be maintained at a pH of 6.2 or higher. They are gently agitated during storage, a move that prevents aggregation and allows for the diffusion of gases. Once pooled, PLTs must be transfused within 4 hours. Whenever a platelet product is entered in a nonsterile manner, it must be transfused within 4 hours.[2,5,16]

Indications

Platelet transfusion is indicated to treat bleeding caused by thrombocytopenia and/or congenital or acquired qualitative platelet dysfunction.[2,5,6,16,49-52] The normal platelet count of a neonate is the same as that of older children and adults. The general indications for platelet transfusion are presented in Table 8. In general, a platelet count of 50,000/µL is considered hemostatic unless the patient has other underlying illnesses.

The indications for platelet transfusion in neonates are presented in Table 9. Premature infants less than 37 weeks with comorbid disease have poor platelet function and decreased levels of plasma coagulation proteins, putting them at greater risk for intracranial hemorrhage. In addition, the underdeveloped subependymal matrix with poorly supported endothelial lining

Table 8. Guidelines for Platelet Transfusion in Older Children*

1. Maintain platelet count ≥100,000/μL for central nervous system (CNS) bleeding or planned CNS surgery.

2. Maintain platelet count ≥50,000/μL if actively bleeding or undergoing major surgery.

3. Prophylactic transfusion for patients with platelet counts between 5 to 10,000/μL.

*Adapted from Roseff, Luban, Manno.[6]

capillaries is predisposed to rupture in the preterm brain.[6,53-55] Because of this increased risk of bleeding, platelet transfusion is generally recommended in a sick premature infant when the platelet count is less than 100,000/μL. Conversely, a stable pre-

Table 9. Guidelines for Platelet Transfusion in Neonates*

1. Platelet count 5000 to 10,000/μL with failure of platelet production

2. Platelet count <30,000/μL in neonate with failure of platelet production

3. Platelet count <50,000/μL in stable premature infant
   - With active bleeding
   - Invasive procedure with failure of platelet production

4. Platelet count <100,000/μL in sick premature infant
   - With active bleeding
   - Invasive procedure in patient with disseminated intravascular coagulation

*Adapted from Roseff, Luban, Manno.[6]

mature infant should be transfused if the platelet count is less than 50,000/μL if there is active bleeding, or if an invasive procedure is planned.[6,53,55-58] Special considerations for neonatal alloimmune thrombocytopenia will be discussed in Alloimmune Cytopenias.

Contraindications and Precautions

Platelet transfusion is not recommended for the treatment of idiopathic thrombocytopenic purpura (ITP), because the same mechanism that causes destruction of autologous platelets can also lead to destruction of transfused platelets. In addition, some patients with ITP have normal bleeding times with adequate hemostasis in the face of thrombocytopenia. Therefore, transfusion should be used only if the patient is actively bleeding. Likewise, platelet transfusion is contraindicated for patients with thrombotic thrombocytopenic purpura/hemolytic-uremic syndrome (TTP/HUS) or heparin-induced thrombocytopenia (HIT), unless there is active bleeding or a planned surgical procedure. These thrombotic diseases can be "fueled" by the administration of platelets. Patients with hypersplenism usually do not have the expected response from platelet transfusion because of splenic sequestration of transfused platelets. Higher doses may be necessary to achieve the desired result.[2,5,6,49-51]

In contrast to red cells and plasma, platelets do not have to be ABO compatible (plasma of the donor compatible with red cells of the recipient), and the use of ABO-incompatible platelets is acceptable practice in larger children under most circumstances. For patients who will receive multiple platelet transfusions (such as those undergoing chemotherapy or marrow transplantation) or will receive larger plasma volume apheresis, it is recommended that ABO-compatible platelets be given because there have been reports of hemolysis in this setting.[2,6,59,60] ABO-incompatible plasma from incompatible platelets can coat the recipient's red cells, causing a positive direct antiglobulin test (DAT).[2,5] Even with a positive DAT, clinically significant hemolysis is rare.[5]

Infants should be transfused with ABO-compatible platelets, whenever possible, because of their small blood volume. If

ABO-compatible platelets are not available, volume reduction can be helpful as a means to remove incompatible plasma, when necessary. Volume reduction requires centrifugation of the component, and there are data that indicate this extra manipulation can lead to platelet activation.[61,62] In the absence of definitive data on its effects on posttransfusion recovery, volume reduction should not be considered routine practice.

Because platelets contain a small amount of red cells, they should be Rh-compatible with the recipient to prevent the development of anti-D in D-negative recipients. However, if D-positive platelets are administered to a D-negative patient, Rh Immune Globulin (RhIG) can be used to prevent immunization. Because one full dose of RhIG can protect the transfusion recipient for up to 15 mL of D-positive red cells, this dose can be used for transfusion of 30 units of D-positive PLTs (each containing about 0.5 mL of red cells) or 7 units of PP (containing about 2 mL of red cells). RhIG is available as either an intramuscular or intravenous preparation. The intravenous form is convenient when high doses of RhIG are necessary, thus avoiding multiple intramuscular injections, or when intramuscular injection would cause injury.[2] Although many institutions offer immune prophylaxis in this setting, it is important to note that the package insert does not address its use in premature infants. In addition, infants under 4 months of age rarely form alloantibodies. When used, RhIG should be administered within 72 hours of exposure, although it may provide protection beyond this time frame.

Dose and Administration

When one calculates the dose of platelets for a child, 5 to 10 mL/kg of either a PLT or PP component should result in a 50,000/µL increase in platelet count (Table 5). For children over 10 kg, a dose of 1 PLT unit per 10 kg should produce similar results.[6,55] This response can be blunted if the infant or child is septic, febrile, or has disseminated intravascular coagulation (DIC) or other evidence of consumptive coagulopathy.[2] For small infants, 1 PLT unit is sufficient. It is important to account for the dead space of the tubing and administration set, which can be considerable

(30 mL or more). Volume reduction of platelet concentrates usually is not necessary, because using the recommended dosages should yield an adequate increase. In addition, centrifugation may cause activation of the platelets, resulting in a less efficacious product, as well as a 33% reduction in recovery.[2]

Platelets should be transfused through a standard 170- to 260-micron blood filter. For the transfusion of a single PLT unit, an 80-micron filter may be used. The smaller filter is ideal for these smaller-volume transfusions because it has less tubing and, therefore, less dead space.

Aliquots

If the blood supplier provides only PP, it may be necessary to prepare aliquots for pediatric transfusion. Bags and syringes used for small-volume RBC transfusion must be used for platelet aliquots because there are no systems specifically designed for platelets.[48] It is important to transfuse the component as soon after dispensing as possible, but no later than 6 hours because the plastic of the bags and syringes does not allow for optimal storage of platelets.[63] Blood manufacturing facilities cannot create aliquots because no systems are approved by the Food and Drug Administration for this purpose. Aliquots must be created in the transfusion service, using a sterile connecting device that splices and reanneals tubing, thus preserving the sterility of the product.[48]

Platelets Leukocytes Reduced

Platelets Leukocytes Reduced can be prepared at the time of manufacturing by the collection facility, in the transfusion service laboratory, or at the bedside. Platelets Pheresis Leukocytes Reduced collected by licensed, automated, apheresis technology are leukocyte reduced during the manufacturing process and contain less than 5×10^6 white cells. When products are leukocyte reduced before storage (by the manufacturer or in the transfusion service), bedside leukocyte reduction filters should not be used because the necessary reduction has been accomplished and further filtration will reduce the number of platelets in the component.[2,16]

Plasma Components

Description of Component

Plasma is usually derived from whole blood donation, when it is separated from whole blood by centrifugation. If it can be frozen within 8 hours of collection using a rapid freezing technique, it is labeled as Fresh Frozen Plasma (FFP). Freezing plasma within 8 hours preserves the labile clotting Factors V and VIII. Larger children and adults require multiple individual units of FFP for a therapeutic dose. Plasma can also be collected using apheresis technology. In this manner, one donor can provide a double product roughly equivalent to 2 units of FFP, referred to as "jumbo plasma." Depending on the required dose, the use of jumbo plasma can reduce donor exposure.[2,5,48] The composition of FFP is found in Table 10.

FFP is stored at –18 C for up to 1 year after its collection. One milliliter contains 1 unit of coagulation factor activity. FFP is typically 200 to 250 mL in volume.[2,5] Because of the rapid freezing that takes place during its production, in the absence of a cryoprotectant agent, white cells are essentially nonfunctional. Therefore, leukocyte reduction and irradiation are unnecessary.

Thawed plasma and plasma frozen within 24 hours have the same properties as FFP, with slightly lower levels of Factor V and Factor VIII. FFP, thawed plasma, and plasma frozen within 24 hours are used to reconstitute whole blood when patients are undergoing exchange transfusion, when whole blood primes are required, and when a patient has multiple factor deficiencies, similar to the uses of FFP. Of note, one small study showed no statistically significant difference in Factor V activity of thawed plasma after 5 days of storage and for Factor VIII at 3 days of storage.[64] Another report showed acceptable recovery of coagulation factors in plasma frozen within 24 hours.[65] These products must be ABO compatible with the red cells used (see Table 4).[2,5]

Indications

The transfusion of FFP is indicated when the patient is bleeding, or when an invasive procedure is planned in a patient with a docu-

Table 10. Coagulation Factors[2]

Factor	Name	In-vivo Half-life	% of Normal Needed for Hemostasis	% In-vivo Recovery	Initial Therapeutic Dose
I	Fibrinogen	3-6 days	12-50	50-70	1-2 bags cryoprecipitate/ 10 kg body weight
II	Prothrombin	2-5 days	10-25	50	10-20 units/kg body weight
V	Labile factor, Proaccelerin	4.5-36 hours	10-30	~80	10-20 mL plasma/kg body weight
VII	Stable factor, Proconvertin	2-5 hours	>10	100	10-20 units/kg body weight
VIII	Antihemophilic factor	8-12 hours	30-40	60-70	10-50 IU/kg, depending on indication
IX	Plasma thromboplastin component, Christmas factor	18-24 hours	15-40	20	20-100 IU/kg, depending on indication
X	Stuart-Prower factor	20-42 hours	10-40	50-95	10-20 units/kg body weight

XI	Plasma thromboplastin antecedent (PTA)	40-80 hours	20-30	90	10-20 mL/kg body weight
XIII	Fibrin stabilizing factor	12 days	<5	50-100	500 mL plasma every 3 weeks
AT	Antithrombin	60-90 hours	80-120	50-100	40-50 IU/kg body weight

Notes:
1. All dosings are provided as a general guideline for initial therapy; the exact loading dose and maintenance intervals should be individualized for each patient.
2. One unit of coagulation factor is present in each mL of fresh frozen plasma.
3. DDAVP is the treatment of choice for patients with hemophilia A who are responders.
4. Composite data from the following references:
   a. Beutler E, Lichtman MA, Coller BS, Kipps TL, eds. Williams' hematology. 5th ed. New York: McGraw-Hill, 1995:1413-58, 1657.
   b. Mollison PL, Engelfriet CP, Contreras M. Blood transfusion in clinical medicine. 10th ed. Oxford: Blackwell Scientific Publications, 1997:459-88.
   c. Huestis DW, Bove JR, Case J, eds. Practical blood transfusion. 4th ed. Boston, MA: Little Brown and Co, 1988:319.
   d. Counts RB, Haisch C, Simon TL, et al. Hemostasis in massively transfused trauma patients. Ann Surg 1979;190:91-9.
   e. Package inserts.

mented coagulation factor deficiency or with a prothrombin time (PT) greater than 1.5 × the midpoint of the age-related normal value, a partial thromboplastin time (PTT) greater than 1.5 × the top of age-related normal values, or both.[49,51] Indications for its use are summarized in Table 11. Because FFP contains all coagulation factors, it is most commonly used in patients with liver disease, DIC with bleeding, and dilutional coagulopathy caused by massive transfusion. The sample for coagulation testing must be obtained from a heparin-free source to ensure that the laboratory values are representative of the patient's ability to form clots. Although it may be difficult to obtain uncontaminated samples, it is essential to avoid plasma transfusion in the absence of clinical need. FFP should be used *only* if a specific factor concentrate is not available, such as Factors V, X, or XI, because individual, single-factor concentrates have usually undergone virus inactivation during the manufacturing process. FFP is indicated for rapid reversal of warfarin when there is bleeding or an anticipated invasive procedure with an international normalized ratio (INR) greater

Table 11. Guidelines for the Transfusion of Fresh Frozen Plasma*

1. Replacement therapy

    - When specific factor concentrates are not available, including but not limited to Factors II, V, X, and XI, protein C or S
    - PT >1.5 × mid-range of age-related normal value and/or PTT >1.5 × top of age-related normal value
    - During therapeutic plasma exchange when FFP is indicated (plasma from which the cryoprecipitate has been removed may be beneficial in thrombotic thrombocytopenic purpura not responsive to conventional plasma exchange)

2. Reversal of warfarin in an emergency situation, such as before an invasive procedure with active bleeding

*Adapted from Roseff, Luban, Manno.[6]
Note: FFP is not indicated for volume expansion or enhancement of wound healing.

than 1.6.[51] Alternatively, vitamin K should be used for warfarin reversal if the situation is not urgent.

For large children and teenagers, a dose of 2.5 to 10 mg vitamin K (up to 25 mg) is expected to control hemorrhage caused by warfarin within 3 to 6 hours, with normalization of the PT seen at 12 to 14 hours. If time permits, it is preferable to use vitamin K, reserving the use of FFP for patients in need of more rapid hemostasis.

FFP is also the replacement fluid used to treat TTP, HUS, or both by plasmapheresis. Cryosupernatant, also referred to as "cryopoor plasma," is used as an alternative to FFP for treating TTP or for patients who are refractory to initial treatment with FFP, because it lacks large-molecular-weight von Willebrand multimers.[66] Cryosupernatant is prepared by removing cryoprecipitate from FFP.[2,5]

The use of FFP to treat DIC is controversial because a component of the disorder is thrombotic. If the need for hemostasis outweighs the need for anticoagulation, FFP transfusion should be used when therapy of the underlying illness has begun and when there is acute bleeding, along with elevations of the PT/PTT as described earlier. FFP should not be used for minor prolongations of PT/PTT because these laboratory values are not usually associated with excessive bleeding.[2,5,6,49,51]

Newborn infants have moderately decreased levels of vitamin-K-dependent clotting factors (Factors II, VII, IX, and X) within the first 48 to 72 hours of birth. The transient decrease, which is most prominent between 2 and 7 days of age, can lead to spontaneous bleeding. In the United States, infants are given a prophylactic dose of 1 mg of intramuscular vitamin K immediately after birth to prevent this decrease and potential hemorrhagic disease of the newborn. Premature infants may require intravenous vitamin K.[67] For infants requiring treatment for other reasons, 1 mg of subcutaneous or intramuscular vitamin K is given as a starting dose, with changes based on clinical needs.

Contraindications and Precautions

FFP is not indicated for volume expansion.[2,6,49,51] Prophylactic use of FFP for volume expansion in infants less than 32 weeks of gestational age has been shown to have no effect on mortality or subsequent disability.[68,69] Patients requiring volume expansion should receive colloids such as albumin, or crystalloids, because these preparations are not associated with the transmission of viral pathogens. Likewise, FFP should not be used as a source of protein for nutritional support; other protein-containing products that do not transmit viral pathogens should be used instead. Because of the transfused plasma proteins, FFP can cause allergic transfusion reactions. Other adverse effects are discussed in Adverse Effects of Blood Transfusion.[2,5,6,49,51]

Dose and Administration

FFP must be ABO compatible with the recipient (see Table 4). FFP is administered in doses of 10 to 15 mL/kg, with an expected 15% to 20% increase in factor levels under conditions of ideal recovery (see Table 5).[2] If FFP has been thawed, it should be used as soon as possible and within 24 hours of thawing. It can be used interchangeably with thawed plasma in all clinical situations because Factors V and VIII levels are maintained above the hemostatic range.[64,65,70] Thawed plasma should be used with caution in patients with consumptive coagulopathy and decreased levels of Factors V and VIII. Using thawed plasma has the advantage of avoiding possible delays while waiting for FFP to be thawed. Because the effects of FFP last approximately 6 to 12 hours, it is important to administer it within the desired time frame to avoid the need for repetitive doses. A standard 180-micron blood filter is used for transfusion. An 80-micron filter can be used for small-volume transfusions.

Aliquots

After FFP is thawed, aliquots can be prepared using a sterile connecting device and transfer bags that are used for red cells aliquots, because no transfer bags are specifically designed for FFP. Some blood centers also manufacture small-volume FFP to use for infants. The plasma collected from one donor can be divided into two or three 75-mL bags that are usually dispensed as a set. Jumbo plasma, although useful to decrease donor exposure in larger children, is impractical and wasteful to use for neonatal transfusion.[6]

Cryoprecipitated Antihemophilic Factor

Description of Component

Cryoprecipitated Antihemophilic Factor (AHF) is prepared by thawing 1 unit of FFP at 1 to 6 C. The supernatant is removed. The remaining precipitate contains concentrated levels of Factor VIII:C (procoagulant activity), Factor XIII, fibrinogen, and Factor VIII:von Willebrand factor (vWF) in a volume of 10 to 15 mL. This concentration is especially important for a small patient. It is stored at –18 C for up to 1 year. The small volume allows more rapid replacement of these specific factors than a single unit of FFP (~ 200 mL) and reduces the risk of volume overload. Each unit of cryoprecipitate contains 80 to 120 units of Factor VIII, at least 150 mg of fibrinogen, 20% to 30% of the original Factor XIII, and 40% to 70% of the original vWF contained in the original unit of FFP.[2,5,16] It is important to note that the contents outlined here represent minimum values, and quality control data from individual blood manufacturers may be higher, with fibrinogen levels typically in the range of 200 to 250 mg.

Indications

Cryoprecipitate is a concentrated source of fibrinogen, Factor VIII, and Factor XIII.[2,5,49,51] Its uses are summarized in Table 12.[6,49,52,71] Despite its high levels of Factor VIII, cryoprecipitate is not the product of choice for treating hemophilia; recombinant or virus-inactivated products remain first-line treatment, with cryoprecipitate being reserved for emergencies when the other products are not available. Likewise, patients with von Willebrand disease should be treated with pharmacologic agents (eg, DDAVP) or virus-inactivated factor concentrates (eg, Humate P, Aventis Behring, King of Prussia, PA) as primary therapy. Platelet dys-

Table 12. Guidelines for the Use of Cryoprecipitate*

1. Hypofibrinogenemia or dysfibrinogenemia with active bleeding or undergoing an invasive procedure
2. Factor XIII deficiency with active bleeding or undergoing an invasive procedure
3. Limited directed donor cryoprecipitate for bleeding episodes in small children with hemophilia A (note that previously untreated children should receive recombinant Factor VIII)
4. von Willebrand disease when DDAVP is contraindicated or not available, and when virus-inactivated plasma-derived Factor VIII concentrate, which contains vWF, is not available
   - Active bleeding
   - Before an invasive procedure

*Adapted from Roseff, Luban, Manno.[6]

function secondary to uremia may respond to transfusion of cryoprecipitate but should be used only if other medical therapies that carry less infectious disease risk are unsuccessful.

Fibrin sealants, composed of virus-inactivated fibrinogen (from cryoprecipitate) that is activated by human thrombin and calcium, have been used during surgery to achieve rapid topical hemostasis and as adhesives.[72-76] These commercially prepared products have greater bonding strength, more rapid preparation time, and increased safety profile resulting from virus inactivation processes during manufacturing, when compared with older preparations made in the operating room. In addition, the older bedside formulations used bovine thrombin. Patients exposed to bovine thrombin are at risk for developing antibodies to bovine Factor V that cross-reacts with human Factor V and can lead to serious hemorrhage. The use of a human source of thrombin prevents this sensitization. There is limited experience with fibrin sealants in the pediatric population.[76] Home-grown preparations of fibrin sealant that combined cryoprecipitate and bovine thrombin directly on the operative site should not be used because of their risk of virus transmission and sensitization to bovine thrombin.

Contraindications and Precautions

Cryoprecipitate should not be used to treat patients with Factor VIII deficiency or von Willebrand disease when other, safer products exist. Because of its small volume, cryoprecipitate does not have to be ABO compatible with the recipient. In high-volume transfusions, though, infusion of ABO-incompatible cryoprecipitate may result in a positive DAT and a risk of hemolysis caused by passive transfer of ABO antibodies. Neonates should be given only ABO-compatible cryoprecipitate because of their small blood volume.[2,5]

Dose and Administration

A dose of 1 to 2 units/10 kg raises a small child's fibrinogen level about 60 to 100 mg/dL (Table 5). In infants, a single unit of cryoprecipitate as a standard dose is usually sufficient to achieve hemostasis. Once cryoprecipitate is pooled, it should be transfused within 4 hours of pooling or 6 hours after thawing, if an individual unit is used. Because of its small volume, cryoprecipitate does not need to be prepared into aliquots for neonatal transfusion.[2,5,48] A standard 180-micron blood filter is used for transfusion. An 80-micron filter may be used for small-volume transfusions of single units.

Granulocytes

Description of Component

Granulocytes are collected from donors by apheresis. Donors may be unstimulated, stimulated with steroids, or, more commonly, stimulated with steroids and granulocyte colony-stimulating factor (G-CSF). Donors who have received G-CSF produce yields about sixfold higher than standard donors, and those donors stimulated with G-CSF while receiving dexamethasone can produce yields almost threefold higher than with G-CSF alone.[3,77] Stimulating donors with pharmacologic agents is not a routine practice at most blood centers. Granulocyte products must contain at least 1×10^{10} granulocytes. Because of the significant red cell content, the products must be ABO compatible with the donor, and a crossmatch is required. In addition, platelets are present in granulocyte products and provide an additional benefit if the patient is also thrombocytopenic. Granulocytes are stored at room temperature, without agitation, and should be used as soon as possible after collection because their viability rapidly declines. They must be infused within 24 hours of collection.[2,5,16,78]

Indications

Any decisions regarding the transfusion of granulocytes should be made in consultation with the transfusion medicine physician because of a lack of established efficacy in randomized controlled trials. Indications for transfusion are summarized in Table 13.[2,6,79] Neonates are at increased risk of bacterial sepsis; premature infants are the most vulnerable. Although neutrophilia is an important part of the host response to fight infection and is used as a sign of sepsis, for the newborn with decreased marrow reserve a decrease in the neutrophil storage pool can result in neutropenia. In

Table 13. Guidelines for Granulocyte Transfusion in Children*

1. Neonates and children with neutropenia or granulocyte dysfunction with bacterial sepsis and lack of responsiveness to standard therapy

2. Neutropenic neonates and children with fungal disease not responsive to standard therapy

*Adapted from Roseff, Luban, Manno.[6]

this setting, granulocytes have been successfully used as an adjunct to antibiotic therapy.[79-82]

For older patients, a trial of granulocyte therapy should be contemplated only in a patient with neutropenia (absolute neutrophil count <500/µL) and documented infection that is unresponsive to standard medical therapy for at least 24 to 48 hours, in the setting of reversible myeloid hypoplasia. There has been speculation that the lack of proven efficacy of granulocytes in large children and adults is due to limitations in collecting a sufficiently high dose. The better response seen using this form of therapy in infants and children is probably due to their smaller blood volume.[2,5,6,78,79]

Contraindications and Precautions

Granulocyte transfusion is a supportive, adjunctive therapy that should be used with other therapies, such as antibiotic use and growth factors, while waiting for marrow recovery. Transfusion of granulocytes is frequently accompanied by chills, fever, and allergic reactions,[78,79] and it should be discontinued in patients who experience severe pulmonary reactions. Granulocyte transfusion and amphotericin administration should be separated by as much time as is practical because severe pulmonary reactions have been reported with concomitant use of amphotericin B, probably the result of enhanced granulocyte aggregation. In a small in-vitro study, a liposomal preparation of amphotericin B caused significantly less granulocyte aggregation, and there is hope that future in-vivo studies will demonstrate its safety as concomitant therapy in patients receiving granulocyte transfusion.[83] Because the human herpes viruses are carried in white cells, there is a risk of cytomegalovirus (CMV) transmission during transfusion, and granulocytes should be collected from CMV-seronegative donors if herpes is a concern. Because granulocytes contain significant numbers of red cells and plasma, they must be ABO identical with the recipient and crossmatch compatible. The risk of alloimmunization to antigens carried on white cells is particularly important to consider in a patient who may be anticipating transplantation. This risk should be taken into account when family members are being considered as sources of progenitor cells; these individuals should not serve as granulocyte donors before the transplantation procedure. Patients who are alloimmunized should receive HLA-matched granulocyte products. Because of the presence of fresh lymphocytes and infusion into an immunocompromised patient, granulocytes must be irradiated using gamma irradiation to prevent transfusion-associated graft-vs-host disease. Granulocytes should be transfused through standard 180-micron blood administration filters but should *not* be administered through leukocyte reduction filters.[2,5,6,50] See Table 14 for a list of requirements for granulocyte products.

Table 14. Requirements for Granulocyte Products Intended for Children

- Ensure ABO compatibility (consider using ABO-identical units for neonates, patients undergoing hematopoietic progenitor cell transplantation, or patients undergoing high-dose chemotherapy for a hematopoietic malignancy)
- Ensure that they are crossmatch compatible
- Irradiate
- Transfuse as soon as possible
- Use standard blood filter
- Do not use leukocyte reduction filter
- Administer within 4 to 6 hours of collection
- Do not administer with amphotericin; separate administration by as much time as practical
- Use HLA-matched components in alloimmunized patients
- Infuse over 1 to 2 hours
- Use CMV-seronegative units if recipient is CMV seronegative

Dose and Administration

For infants, a dose of 10 to 15 mL/kg is recommended, which should deliver 1×10^9 to 2×10^9 PMN/kg.[55,79] Because neonatal neutrophil function is often abnormal, the use of granulocyte transfusions in this age group is beneficial.[55,78-82] The efficacy of granulocyte transfusion in neonates appears to be dose dependent, with doses greater than 1×10^9 PMN/kg offering better clinical response. Granulocyte concentrates prepared by apheresis produce a higher yield than those produced from buffy coats.[81] For adults and larger children, a dose of at least 1×10^{10} PMN/kg is recommended.[2,81] The logistics of granulocyte collection must be carefully arranged with the local blood collection facility and the hospital's transfusion service. It is important to plan for multiple donors because these components are usually administered daily for 5 or more consecutive days. Because the components must be used in less than 24 hours, it is important to recognize that infectious disease testing may not be completed before the component is used. The risks and benefits of transfusing an untested component must be weighed by the transfusing physician in conjunction with the patient's parents. Some blood collection facilities attempt to obtain granulocytes from frequent platelet donors who have been tested recently and found acceptable for donation. On other occasions, a granulocyte donor may be asked to submit a blood sample for testing before collection and, if negative for all infectious disease markers, to serve as a donor. Obtaining blood from donors who are stimulated with growth factors before donation also requires careful coordination.[2,6]

Granulocytes should be transfused over 1 to 2 hours as tolerated. If the patient develops a transfusion reaction, he or she can be treated with antipyretics and steroids. Meperidine can be used to treat rigors. As a result of the rapid degradation of granulocytes in storage, as well as the importance of delivering the highest possible dose, the largest volume that can be tolerated by the patient should be administered as soon as possible.[2,78] The dose should not be split, which means that the rest of the unit would be given when the component is not as efficacious.

Whole Blood

In general, Whole Blood transfusions offer no significant medical benefits over blood component transfusions. Indeed, most hospitals do not use Whole Blood, and most blood centers will produce Whole Blood only when specifically ordered. The contents of Whole Blood are included in Table 1.[2,5,6]

One controversial study suggests that Whole Blood is indicated for patients who are less than 2 years old and who undergo certain complex cardiac surgeries and require cardiopulmonary bypass. The data showed that such patients bleed less following surgery if they are transfused with 1 unit of fresh Whole Blood (less than 48 hours old) immediately following cardiopulmonary bypass.[84] Results of platelet aggregation studies suggested that the hemostatic benefit in this patient population was due to superior platelet function following Whole Blood transfusion. However, this benefit has not been seen in other patient populations. Furthermore, Whole Blood is stored at 1 to 6 C, and platelets stored at this temperature are rapidly cleared by the reticuloendothelial system because of irreversible aggregation of the vWF receptors on platelet membranes.[85,86]

Donor-Specific Units

Autologous Red Blood Cells

Autologous blood is blood that has been collected from the patient for reinfusion in a planned, perioperative setting. Blood can be collected before the date of surgery (preoperative), at the initiation of surgery (acute normovolemic hemodilution), or during surgery (perioperative recovery). In the setting of neonatal transfusion, umbilical cord blood collected at the time of birth or cord blood infused during delayed clamping of the umbilical cord can also be considered forms of autologous transfusion. The major advantages of autologous donation are decreased risks of viral infection and immunologic exposure posed by allogeneic transfusion. Autologous blood can serve as a source of compatible blood for later use by patients immunized with multiple antibodies. Autologous blood should be ordered only for children who can safely donate blood for themselves and when there is a high likelihood of transfusion.[2,6,53]

Many studies document the safety of preoperative autologous donation in children. Autologous transfusion has been shown to be effective in markedly decreasing allogeneic blood exposure in infants and children from as early as 3 months of age.[2,6,53,87-90] It is essential to weigh the risks and benefits of autologous donation when deciding whether to proceed with this option in young children. The risks of autologous donation in adults, such as lowering presurgical hemoglobin and occult bacteremia in the presurgical patient leading to life-threatening septic transfusion reactions, are well documented.[91-93]

Infants and small children bring additional issues to the decision and represent a different group of autologous donors and patients. In contrast to volunteer adult donors who must weigh at least 110 lbs, pediatric autologous blood donors may have smaller blood volumes with a decreased ability to compensate for volume changes. In addition, they may not be able to cooperate with the donation process, requiring sedation, which has attendant risks. Logistically, most donation sets have 16-gauge needles that are too large for small veins, and venous access can be challenging. A sterile connecting device can be used to attach smaller needles, from 17 to 20 gauge, realizing that the smaller the needle, the greater the risk for hemolysis. The amount of anticoagulant in the collection set must be adjusted for the smaller-volume donor by using a sterile connecting device to withdraw excess anticoagulant. Informed consent must be obtained from the patient's parents.[2,6,53,87-90]

Perioperative blood recovery has not been explored fully in children. Limited studies have shown that such procedures are safe in the pediatric population and that they can decrease the use of allogeneic blood components. Contraindications to collecting blood intraoperatively include gross contamination of the operative field with bacteria, tumor, or both.[2,6,94,95]

Some studies have shown that blood collected from the umbilical cord at the time of delivery and later transfused may decrease allogeneic blood exposure.[2,5,96-98] Unfortunately, only 75 to 125 mL of blood can usually be collected, with the smallest infants who have the greatest needs yielding the smallest collection volumes. There has been concern about bacterial contamination of cord blood and no comparisons exist between banked allogeneic blood and cord blood with respect to efficacy and quality.[98,99] One alternative for infants without volume constraints who need additional oxygen-carrying capacity is a generous placental-fetal transfusion at the time of delivery.[53,100]

Directed Blood Donations

Directed donor blood is donated by family or friends of the patient. Many blood banks provide this service despite the increased administrative cost for a practice that has no additional therapeutic benefit over blood from other volunteer donors. A directed donor component must be compatible with the patient. Additionally, although directed donors must pass the same screening requirements as community volunteer blood donors, a small increased risk of infectious disease transmission may exist because these donors might feel pressured to donate and may fail to reveal risky behaviors at the time of donation. Indeed, directed donors tend to have a higher incidence of positive tests for infectious disease markers than the general volunteer blood donors and may be less safe.[101-104]

The risk of transfusion-associated graft-vs-host disease is increased if the directed blood donor is genetically related to the patient. To prevent this risk, cellular blood components from blood relatives should be irradiated before transfusion; many transfusion services irradiate all blood from directed donors.[2]

An additional risk is associated with directed donations from relatives to patients who may require a hematopoietic progenitor cell transplant. Transfusions can induce antibodies to donor HLA antigens. If the blood donor is a genetic relative, then the transfusion-induced HLA antibodies may be directed against antigens that are expressed by cells of potential hematopoietic progenitor cell donors. However, when family members are the best possible donors, leukocyte reduction of cellular components from directed donors reduces the likelihood of HLA-antibody formation.

In some scenarios, cellular blood components from directed donors can be medically advantageous. For patients with multiple antibodies or those with an antibody to a high-frequency antigen, such as the HPA-1a antibody that usually causes neonatal alloimmune thrombocytopenia in Caucasians,[105,106] family members may be the only way to get compatible blood components quickly.

Neonates

Directed donations from parents are safe for many children, including neonates.[107] However, directed donations from parents are a poor choice for some neonates who have immune-mediated hemolysis or thrombocytopenia. These immunologic conditions usually occur when the neonatal circulation contains maternal antibodies directed against paternally inherited antigens. Maternal blood components that contain plasma should be used with caution because they may contain antibodies to antigens on the child's cells, and these transfused antibodies may exacerbate hemolysis or thrombocytopenia.[108] Paternal cellular blood components may be a poor choice for these neonates because the maternal antibodies are directed against antigens inherited from the father, and these antigens are expressed on transfused paternal cells.[108]

Component Therapy for Patients Undergoing Extracorporeal Membrane Oxygenation

ECMO is a form of cardiopulmonary bypass used to support patients with reversible pulmonary disease or temporary cardiac insufficiency, accomplished through either venoarterial or venovenous access. Standard guidelines for transfusion of blood components for patients undergoing ECMO do not exist, and protocols can vary depending on the type of circuit being used. To prevent thrombosis and platelet activation in the circuitry and extensive tubing, patients are heparinized, resulting in a significant risk of bleeding.[2,6,109]

It is important that the members of the ECMO team communicate with the transfusion service, so that the logistics are prearranged and the infant's needs are met without delays.[109] Most programs have standard orders that include the prime, usually 2 to 3 RBC units (not washed), depending on the infant's size, and 1 unit of FFP. Platelet counts are maintained between 80,000 and 150,000/µL, with the upper limit of this range sometimes reserved for infants who are actively bleeding. Likewise, hemoglobin levels are variable but usually are maintained between 10 and 12 g/dL. Coagulation is frequently monitored by activated clotting times due to the presence of heparin that can alter other laboratory measures of coagulation. FFP and cryoprecipitate are used for replacement of clotting factors. Algorithms for replacement are variable.[109,110]

It is generally recommended that red cells used during ECMO be less than 7 to 14 days old, because the process is akin to a massive transfusion. The increased potassium contained in large volumes of blood more than 7 days old can be clinically significant for infants who have undergone cardiac surgery.[109] A recent abstract reported that using red cells preserved in AS1 and AS3 was safe and efficacious during ECMO.[111] Mounting anecdotal experience leads to the same conclusion. For centers concerned about additives, red cells preserved in CPD, CP2D, or CPDA-1 may be used.

References

1. Rudolph CD. Rudolph's pediatrics. 21st ed. New York: McGraw-Hill, 2003.
2. Brecher ME, ed. Technical manual. 14th ed. Bethesda, MD: American Association of Blood Banks, 2002.
3. Stroncek DF, Yau YY, Oblitas J, Leitman SF. Administration of G-CSF plus dexamethasone produces greater gran-

ulocyte concentrate yields while causing no more donor toxicity than G-CSF alone. Transfusion 2001;41:1037-44.
4. Dale DC, Liles WC, Llewellyn C, et al. Neutrophil transfusions: Kinetics and functions of neutrophils mobilized with granulocyte-colony-stimulating factor and dexamethasone. Transfusion 1998;38:713-21.
5. Triulzi DJ, ed. Blood transfusion therapy: A physician's handbook. 7th ed. Bethesda, MD: American Association of Blood Banks, 2002.
6. Roseff SD, Luban NL, Manno CS. Guidelines for assessing appropriateness of pediatric transfusion. Transfusion 2002;42:1398-413.
7. AuBuchon JP, ed. Guidelines for blood utilization review. Bethesda, MD: American Association of Blood Banks, 2001.
8. Brugnara C, Platt OS. The neonatal erythrocyte and its disorders. In: Nathan DG, Orkin SH, eds. Nathan and Oski's hematology of infancy and childhood. 5th ed. Philadelphia: WB Saunders, 1998:19-52.
9. Voak D, Cann R, Finney RD, et al. Guidelines for administration of blood products: Transfusion of infants and neonates. British Committee for Standards in Haematology Blood Transfusion Task Force. Transfus Med 1994;4:63-9.
10. Fetus and Newborn Committee CPS. Guidelines for transfusion of erythrocytes to neonates and premature infants. Can Med Assoc J 1992;147:1781-92.
11. Wardrop CA, Holland BM, Veale KE, et al. Nonphysiological anaemia of prematurity. Arch Dis Child 1978;53:855-60.
12. Dallman PR. Anemia of prematurity. Annu Rev Med 1981;32:143-60.
13. Doyle JJ. The role of erythropoietin in the anemia of prematurity. Semin Perinatol 1997;21:20-7.
14. Lo L, Singer ST. Thalassemia: Current approach to an old disease. Pediatr Clin North Am 2002;49:1165-91.
15. Montoya AF. Neocyte transfusion: A current perspective. Transfus Sci 1993;14:147-56.

16. Fridey JL, ed. Standards for blood banks and transfusion services. 22nd ed. Bethesda, MD: American Association of Blood Banks, 2003.
17. Sazama K, ed. Accreditation requirements manual. 6th ed. Bethesda, MD: American Association of Blood Banks, 1995.
18. Strauss RG. Additive solutions and product age in neonatal red blood cell transfusion. In: Herman JH, Manno CS, eds. Pediatric transfusion therapy. Bethesda, MD: AABB Press, 2002:129-45.
19. Strauss RG, Burmeister LF, Johnson K, et al. AS-1 red cells for neonatal transfusions: A randomized trial assessing donor exposure and safety. Transfusion 1996;36:873-8.
20. Luban NL, Strauss RG, Hume HA. Commentary on the safety of red cells preserved in extended-storage media for neonatal transfusions. Transfusion 1991;31:229-35.
21. Brecher ME. Collected questions and answers. 6th ed. Bethesda, MD: American Association of Blood Banks, 2000:73-5.
22. Tuchschmid P, Mieth D, Burger R, Duc G. Potential hazard of hypoalbuminemia in newborn babies after exchange transfusions with ADSOL red blood cell concentrates. Pediatrics 1990;85:234-5.
23. Hilsenrath P, Nemechek J, Widness JA, et al. Cost-effectiveness of a limited-donor blood program for neonatal red cell transfusions. Transfusion 1999;39:938-43.
24. Liu EA, Mannino FL, Lane TA. Prospective, randomized trial of the safety and efficacy of a limited donor exposure transfusion program for premature neonates. J Pediatr 1994;125:92-6.
25. Wood A, Wilson N, Skacel P, et al. Reducing donor exposure in preterm infants requiring multiple blood transfusions. Arch Dis Child Fetal Neonatal Ed 1995;72:F29-33.
26. Meryman HT, Hornblower M. The preparation of red cells depleted of leukocytes. Review and evaluation. Transfusion 1986;26:101-6.
27. Sirchia G, Rebulla P, Parravicini A, et al. Leukocyte depletion of red cell units at the bedside by transfusion through a new filter. Transfusion 1987;27:402-5.

28. Federowicz I, Barrett BB, Andersen JW, et al. Characterization of reactions after transfusion of cellular blood components that are white cell reduced before storage. Transfusion 1996;36:21-8.
29. Dzik S. Prestorage leukocyte reduction of cellular blood components. Transfus Sci 1994;15:131-9.
30. Blajchman MA. Immunomodulation and blood transfusion. Am J Ther 2002;9:389-95.
31. Strauss RG. Selection of white cell-reduced blood components for transfusions during early infancy. Transfusion 1993;33:352-7.
32. Wang-Rodriguez J, Fry E, Fiebig E, et al. Immune response to blood transfusion in very-low-birthweight infants. Transfusion 2000;40:25-34.
33. Hillyer CD, Tiegerman KO, Berkman EM. Evaluation of the red cell storage lesion after irradiation in filtered packed red cell units. Transfusion 1991;31:497-9.
34. Brugnara C, Churchill WH. Effect of irradiation on red cell cation content and transport. Transfusion 1992;32:246-52.
35. Moroff G, Holme S, AuBuchon JP, et al. Viability and in vitro properties of AS-1 red cells after gamma irradiation. Transfusion 1999;39:128-34.
36. Van Damme-Lombaerts R, Broyer M, Businger J, et al. A study of recombinant human erythropoietin in the treatment of anaemia of chronic renal failure in children on haemodialysis. Pediatr Nephrol 1994;8:338-42.
37. Bolonaki I, Stiakaki E, Lydaki E, et al. Treatment with recombinant human erythropoietin in children with malignancies. Pediatr Hematol Oncol 1996;13:111-21.
38. Leon P, Jimenez M, Barona P, Sierrasesumaga L. Recombinant human erythropoietin for the treatment of anemia in children with solid malignant tumors. Med Pediatr Oncol 1998;30:110-16.
39. Klaesson S, Ringden O, Ljungman P, et al. Reduced blood transfusions requirements after allogeneic bone marrow transplantation: Results of a randomised, double-blind study with high-dose erythropoietin. Bone Marrow Transplant 1994;13:397-402.

40. Locatelli F, Zecca M, Pedrazzoli P, et al. Use of recombinant human erythropoietin after bone marrow transplantation in pediatric patients with acute leukemia: Effect on erythroid repopulation in autologous versus allogeneic transplants. Bone Marrow Transplant 1994;13:403-10.
41. Parsons SK. Oncology practice patterns in the use of hematopoietic growth factors. Curr Opin Pediatr 2000; 12:10-17.
42. Ohls RK, Ehrenkranz RA, Wright LL, et al. Effects of early erythropoietin therapy on the transfusion requirements of preterm infants below 1250 grams birth weight: A multicenter, randomized, controlled trial. Pediatrics 2001;108:934-42.
43. Donato H, Vain N, Rendo P, et al. Effect of early versus late administration of human recombinant erythropoietin on transfusion requirements in premature infants: Results of a randomized, placebo-controlled, multicenter trial. Pediatrics 2000;105:1066-72.
44. Al-Kharfy T, Smyth JA, Wadsworth L, et al. Erythropoietin therapy in neonates at risk of having bronchopulmonary dysplasia and requiring multiple transfusions. J Pediatr 1996;129:89-96.
45. Shannon KM, Keith JF III, Mentzer WC, et al. Recombinant human erythropoietin stimulates erythropoiesis and reduces erythrocyte transfusions in very low birth weight preterm infants. Pediatrics 1995;95:1-8.
46. Casadevall N, Nataf J, Viron B, et al. Pure red-cell aplasia and antierythropoietin antibodies in patients treated with recombinant erythropoietin. N Engl J Med 2002;346:469-75.
47. Feusner J, Hastings C. Recombinant human erythropoietin in pediatric oncology: A review. Med Pediatr Oncol 2002; 39:463-8.
48. Roseff SD. Pediatric blood collection and transfusion technology. In: Herman JH, Manno CS, eds. Pediatric transfusion therapy. Bethesda, MD: AABB Press, 2002: 217-48.
49. Practice guidelines for blood component therapy: A report by the American Society of Anesthesiologists Task Force

on Blood Component Therapy. Anesthesiology 1996;84:732-47.
50. Consensus conference. Platelet transfusion therapy. JAMA 1987;257:1777-80.
51. Fresh-Frozen Plasma, Cryoprecipitate, and Platelets Administration Practice Guidelines Development Task Force of the College of American Pathologists. Practice parameter for the use of fresh-frozen plasma, cryoprecipitate, and platelets. JAMA 1994;270:777-81.
52. Beutler E. Platelet transfusions: The 20,000/µL trigger. Blood 1993;81:1411-13.
53. Hume HA. Blood components: Preparation, indications and administration. In: Lilleyman JS, Hann IM, Blanchette VS, eds. Pediatric hematology. London: Churchill Livingstone, 1999:709-39.
54. Sacher RA, Luban NL, Strauss RG. Current practice and guidelines for the transfusion of cellular blood components in the newborn. Transfus Med Rev 1989;3:39-54.
55. Strauss RG. Transfusion therapy for neonates. Am J Dis Child 1991;145:904-11.
56. Andrew M, Vegh P, Caco C. A randomized, controlled trial of platelet transfusions in thrombocytopenic premature infants. J Pediatr 1993;123:285-91.
57. Andrew M, Castle V, Saigal S. Clinical impact of neonatal thrombocytopenia. J Pediatr 1987;110:457-64.
58. Castle V, Andrew M, Kelton J. Frequency and mechanism of neonatal thrombocytopenia. J Pediatr 1986;108:749-55.
59. Larsson LG, Welsh VJ, Ladd DJ. Acute intravascular hemolysis secondary to out-of-group platelet transfusion. Transfusion 2000;40:902-6.
60. McManigal S, Sims KL. Intravascular hemolysis secondary to ABO incompatible platelet products. An underrecognized transfusion reaction. Am J Clin Pathol 1999;111:202-6.
61. Holme S, Sweeney JD, Sawyer S, Elfath MD. The expression of p-selectin during collection, processing, and storage of platelet concentrates: Relationship to loss of in vivo viability. Transfusion 1997;37:12-17.

62. Pineda AA, Zylstra VW, Clare DE. Viability and functional integrity of washed platelets. Transfusion 1989; 29:524-7.
63. Pisciotto PT, Snyder EL, Napychank PA, Hopfer SM. In vitro characteristics of volume-reduced platelet concentrate stored in syringes. Transfusion 1991;31:404-8.
64. Downes KA, Wilson E, Yomtovian R, Sarode R. Serial measurement of clotting factors in thawed plasma stored for 5 days (letter). Transfusion 2001;41:570.
65. Smith J, Ness PM, Moroff G, Luban NL. Retention of coagulation factors in plasma, frozen within 24 hours after phlebotomy. Transfusion 1993;33(Suppl):S33.
66. Byrnes JJ, Moake JL, Klug P, Periman P. Effectiveness of the cryosupernatant fraction of plasma in the treatment of refractory thrombotic thrombocytopenic purpura. Am J Hematol 1990;34:169-74.
67. Behrman RE, Kliegman RM, Jensen HB. Nelson textbook of pediatrics. 16th ed. Philadelphia: WB Saunders, 2000.
68. Northern Neonatal Nursing Initiative [NNNI] Trial Group. A randomized trial comparing the effect of prophylactic intravenous fresh frozen plasma, gelatin or glucose on early mortality and morbidity in preterm babies. Eur J Pediatr 1996;155:580-8.
69. Northern Neonatal Nursing Initiative [NNNI] Trial Group. Randomised trial of prophylactic early fresh-frozen plasma or gelatin or glucose in preterm babies: Outcome at 2 years. Lancet 1996;348:229-32.
70. Becker JL, Southers M, Sabau J, Fisher LM. Can the expiration of thawed FFP be extended? (abstract) Transfusion 1999;39:S96P.
71. Krundieck R, Shaw DR, Huang ST. Hemorrhagic disorder due to an isoniazid associated acquired factor XIII inhibitor in a patient with Waldenstrom's macroglobulinemia. Am J Med 1991;90:639-45.
72. Reiner AP. Fibrin glue increasingly popular for topical surgical hemostasis. Lab Med 1999;30:189-93.
73. Alving BM, Weinstein MJ, Finlayson JS, et al. Fibrin sealant: Summary of a conference on characteristics and clinical uses. Transfusion 1995;35:783-90.

74. Radosevich M, Goubran HI, Burnouf T. Fibrin sealant: Scientific rationale, production methods, properties, and current clinical use. Vox Sang 1997;72:133-43.
75. Dadeya S, Ms K. Strabismus surgery: Fibrin glue versus vicryl for conjunctival closure. Acta Ophthalmol Scand 2001;79:515-7.
76. Ortel TL, Mercer MC, Thames EH, et al. Immunologic impact and clinical outcomes after surgical exposure to bovine thrombin. Ann Surg 2001;233:88-96.
77. Bensinger WI, Price TH, Dale DC. The effects of daily recombinant human granulocyte colony-stimulating factor administration on normal granulocyte donors undergoing leukapheresis. Blood 1993;81:1883-8.
78. McCullough J. Granulocyte transfusion. In: Petz LD, Swisher SN, Kleinman S, et al, eds. Clinical practice of transfusion medicine. 3rd ed. New York: Churchill Livingstone, 1996:413-32.
79. Stauss SG. Current issues in neonatal transfusion. Vox Sang 1986;51:1-9.
80. Christensen RD, Bradley PP, Rothstein G. The leukocyte left shift in clinical and experimental neonatal sepsis. J Pediatr 1981;98:101-5.
81. Vamvakas EC, Pineda AA. Meta-analysis of clinical studies of the efficacy of granulocyte transfusions in the treatment of bacterial sepsis. J Clin Apheresis 1996;11:1-9.
82. Cairo MS, Rucker R, Bennetts GA, et al. Improved survival of newborns receiving leukocyte transfusions for sepsis. Pediatrics 1984;74:887-92.
83. Sulis ML, Van de Ven C, Henderson T, et al. Liposomal amphotericin B (AmBisome) compared with amphotericin B ± FMLP induces significantly less in vitro neutrophil aggregation with granulocyte-colony-stimulating factor/dexamethasone-mobilized allogeneic donor neutrophils. Blood 2002;99:384-6.
84. Manno CS, Hedberg KW, Kim HC, et al. Comparison of the hemostatic effects of fresh whole blood, stored whole blood, and components after open heart surgery in children. Blood 1991;77:930-6.

85. Becker GA, Tuccelli M, Kunicki T, et al. Studies of platelet concentrates stored at 22 C and 4 C. Transfusion 1973; 13:61-8.
86. Hoffmeister KM, Felbinger TW, Falet H, et al. The clearance mechanism of chilled blood platelets. Cell 2003; 112:87-97.
87. Thompson HW, Luban NL. Autologous blood transfusion in the pediatric patient. J Pediatr Surg 1995;30:1406-11.
88. Etchason J, Petz L, Keeler E, et al. The cost effectiveness of preoperative autologous blood donations. N Engl J Med 1995;332:719-24.
89. Novak RW. Autologous blood transfusion in a pediatric population. Safety and efficacy. Clin Pediatr (Phila) 1988; 27:184-7.
90. Silvergleid AJ. Safety and effectiveness of predeposit autologous transfusions in preteen and adolescent children. JAMA 1987;257:3403-4.
91. Goodnough LT, Brecher ME, Kanter MH, AuBuchon JP. Transfusion medicine. Second of two parts—blood conservation. N Engl J Med 1999;340:525-33.
92. Cohen JA, Brecher ME. Preoperative autologous blood donation: Benefit or detriment? A mathematical analysis. Transfusion 1995;35:640-4.
93. AuBuchon JP, Birkmeyer JD. Controversies in transfusion medicine. Is autologous blood transfusion worth the cost? Con. Transfusion 1994;34:79-83.
94. Dahmani S, Orliaguet GA, Meyer PG, et al. Perioperative blood salvage during surgical correction of craniosynostosis in infants. Br J Anaesth 2000;85:550-5.
95. Spain DA, Miller FB, Bergamini TM, et al. Quality assessment of intraoperative blood salvage and autotransfusion. Am Surg 1997;63:1059-63, discussion 1063-4.
96. Ballin A, Arbel E, Kenet G, et al. Autologous umbilical cord blood transfusion. Arch Dis Child Fetal Neonatal Ed 1995;73:F181-3.
97. Eichler H, Schaible T, Richter E, et al. Cord blood as a source of autologous RBCs for transfusion to preterm infants. Transfusion 2000;40:1111-17.

98. Surbek DV, Glanzmann R, Senn HP, et al. Can cord blood be used for autologous transfusion in preterm neonates? Eur J Pediatr 2000;159:790-1.
99. Strauss RG. Autologous transfusions for neonates using placental blood. A cautionary note. Am J Dis Child 1992;146:21-2.
100. Kinmond S, Aitchison TC, Holland BM, et al. Umbilical cord clamping and preterm infants: A randomised trial. Br Med J 1993;306(6871):172-5.
101. Starkey JM, MacPherson JL, Bolgiano DC, et al. Markers for transfusion-transmitted disease in different groups of blood donors. JAMA 1989;262:3452-4.
102. Wong ED, Baxter CA, Frey C. Transfusion transmitted viral disease and deferral rates in parental, directed, and community donors for pediatric transfusion (abstract). Transfusion 2001;41(Suppl):114S.
103. Pink J, Thomson A, Wylie B. Infectious disease markers in autologous and directed donations. Transfus Med 1994;4:135-8.
104. Yomtovian R. Is directed blood transfusion a good idea? MLO Med Lab Obs 1992;24:31-4.
105. Spencer JA, Burrows RF. Feto-maternal alloimmune thrombocytopenia: A literature review and statistical analysis. Aust N Z J Obstet Gynaecol 2001;41:45-55.
106. Murphy MF, Williamson LM. Antenatal screening for fetomaternal alloimmune thrombocytopenia: An evaluation using the criteria of the UK National Screening Committee. Br J Haematol 2000;111:726-32.
107. Strauss RG, Burmeister LF, Johnson K, et al. Randomized trial assessing the feasibility and safety of biologic parents as RBC donors for their preterm infants. Transfusion 2000;40:450-6.
108. Elbert C, Strauss RG, Barrett F, et al. Biological mothers may be dangerous blood donors for their neonates. Acta Haematol 1991;85:189-91.
109. Meliones JN, Hansell DR. Extracorporeal membrane oxygenation: The role of blood components. In: Chambers LA, Issitt LA, eds. Supporting the pediatric transfusion re-

cipient. Bethesda, MD: American Association of Blood Banks, 1994:87-107.
110. Minifee PK, Daeschner CW III, Griffin MP, et al. Decreasing blood donor exposure in neonates on extracorporeal membrane oxygenation. J Pediatr Surg 1990;25:38-42.
111. Eder AF, Gray K, Manno CS. Comparison of CPDA with AS red cell transfusion to infants undergoing ECMO (abstract). Am J Clin Pathol 2002;118:628.

ALLOIMMUNE CYTOPENIAS

Overview of Alloimmune Cytopenias

Alloimmune cytopenias result from the antibody-mediated destruction of red cells, platelets, or granulocytes. Infants may be affected before birth or in the neonatal period by maternal antibodies that cross the placenta during pregnancy to cause hemolytic disease, thrombocytopenia, or neutropenia. Children are at risk of active alloimmunization with repeated blood transfusions that may lead to hemolytic destruction of transfused red cells or refractoriness to platelet transfusion. Finally, passively transferred (passenger) lymphocytes following hematopoietic or organ transplantation may cause immune hemolysis in susceptible recipients. Transfusion therapy must be tailored to each of these clinical scenarios encountered in pediatrics.

Immune-Mediated Hemolytic Disease of the Fetus and Newborn

Pathogenesis

Maternal alloantibodies directed against fetal red cell antigens arise following incompatible red cell exposure during pregnancy or transfusion.[1] A vast array of red cell alloantibodies have been implicated in hemolytic disease of the fetus and newborn (HDF/HDN), but most cases of severe fetal anemia that require treatment in utero are caused by anti-D or anti-c (Rhesus), anti-K1 (Kell), or anti-Fy^a (Duffy) (see Table 15).[2,3] ABO IgG isohemagglutinins, which occur without a prior red cell stimulus such as anti-A, anti-B, or anti-A,B, may cause hemolytic disease after birth but do not endanger the fetus. Other predominantly IgM red cell antibodies against carbohydrate blood group antigens (eg, Lewis, P1) do not cross the placenta and are inconsequential in pregnancy.

The likelihood that the fetus will inherit a paternal red cell antigen that its mother lacks depends on the frequency of the blood group alleles in the population.[1] Among Caucasians and African-Americans in the United States, incompatibility with respect to the D antigen occurs in about 10% of all pregnancies; 60% to 70% of D-negative women will have a D-positive infant. In contrast, only 10% of K1-negative women will have a K1-positive infant. Before routine Rh Immune Globulin (RhIG) prophylaxis in obstetric practice, about 15% of D-negative women developed anti-D with childbirth.[4] Anti-D is still one of the most common antibodies associated with HDF/HDN, occurring in about one of 1000 total births, although the rate has dramatically diminished since the introduction of RhIG after 1968.[5] No measures are commercially available to prevent sensitization to other Rhesus antigens or other blood group systems, and these red cell alloantibodies occur in less than 1% of women.[6] Anti-K1 recently surpassed anti-D, being detected at a rate of 3.2 compared to 2.6 per 1000 samples from women, and anti-K1 and other alloantibodies now account for proportionately more cases of HDF/HDN than anti-D (see Table 15).[3,6] Overall, only 16 infant deaths were attributed to alloimmune hemolytic disease of the newborn in the United States in 1999.[7] These statistics accurately reflect the impressive decline in incidence of anti-D, but underestimate the current burden of HDF/HDN because early intrauterine deaths are not captured and neonatal deaths may be attributed to other prevailing complications.

HDF/HDN results from the extravascular destruction of IgG-coated fetal cells in the spleen and reticuloendothelial system. K1 antibodies also suppress erythropoiesis in affected fetuses and newborns.[8] Compensatory hematopoiesis in the marrow and extramedullary hematopoiesis primarily in the liver and spleen result in the release of nucleated red cells, reticulocytes, normoblasts, and other immature erythrocytes in the fetal circulation.

Table 15. HDF/HDN and Blood Groups[2,6,9,10]

Blood Group System	Antibody	Frequency Among Women (per 1000 samples)	Severity of HDF/HDN (Distribution Among Susceptible* Infants)	
ABO	A, B, A,B	~50.0	Not a cause of HDF	
			HDN: None (antibody only):	90%
			Mild/moderate HDN:	<10%
			Severe HDN:	<1%
Rhesus (Rh)	D	2.6	None/mild:	50%
			Moderate:	30%
			Severe:	20%
	c	0.9	None/mild:	70%
			Moderate:	23%
			Severe:	7%
	C	0.7	None/mild:	70-90%
	E	2.0	Rare cases of severe HDF	
	e	Rare		
Lewis	Le^a, Le^b	3.0	Not a cause of HDF/HDN	
Kell	K1	3.2	None/mild:	30%
			Moderate:	30%
			Severe:	38%
Duffy	Fy^a	0.8	None/mild:	94%
			Moderate:	2%
			Severe:	4%
	Fy^b	Rare	Not a cause of HDF/HDN	

(continued)

Table 15. HDF/HDN and Blood Groups[2,6,9,10] (continued)

Blood Group System	Antibody	Frequency Among Women (per 1000 samples)	Severity of HDF/HDN (Distribution Among Susceptible* Infants)
Kidd	Jk^a	0.2	Rare cases of severe HDF
MNSs	M	0.5	Rare cases of severe HDF
	S	0.1	
	U	Rare	
	N	0.03	Not a cause of HDF/HDN
P	P1	0.03	Not a cause of HDF/HDN
Bennett-Goodspeed (HLA)	Bg^a Bg^b Bg^c	Rare	Not a cause of HDF/HDN

*Among women with red cell alloantibodies, susceptible fetuses are those who are antigen- or DAT-positive.

None/mild = no treatment or phototherapy only; moderate = phototherapy and/or neonatal exchange transfusion; severe = hydrops fetalis, intrauterine transfusion, or perinatal death; HDF = hemolytic disease of the fetus; HDN = hemolytic disease of the newborn.

Severe anemia and impaired hepatic function may ultimately lead to hydrops fetalis, which is characterized by generalized edema (anasarca), massive ascites, heart failure, and pleural and pericardial effusions. Immune-mediated destruction of fetal red cells also increases serum unconjugated (indirect) bilirubin. During gestation, unconjugated bilirubin and other metabolites are transported across the placenta and eliminated by the mother. After birth, however, full-term infants are not capable of efficiently metabolizing bilirubin because of their immature liver function and are at risk of developing bilirubin encephalopathy or kernicterus. A premature infant is at greater risk of hyperbilirubinemia and neurologic damage than is a full-term infant as a result of more pronounced liver deficiency and an immature blood-brain barrier.

Clinical Features

About half of Rh-positive infants with detectable maternal anti-D are unaffected or only mildly affected and require no treatment; whereas, 20% are severely affected in utero (Table 15).[2] About half of these severely affected fetuses have significant hemolysis before 34 weeks' gestation and require intrauterine transfusion.[2] A similar spectrum of disease severity is observed with anti-c, anti-K1, and anti-Fy[a], with severe disease affecting 7%, 38%, and 4% of susceptible fetuses, respectively (see Table 15).[2,9,10] On rare occasions, moderate to life-threatening hemolytic disease is caused by various blood group antibodies of different Rhesus, Kidd (anti-Jk[a]), or other red cell specificities.[2,3] First-born infants are usually not affected by maternal red cell alloimmunization and demonstrate only mild HDF/HDN, which reflects the likelihood that significant fetomaternal hemorrhage (FMH) occurs late in the third trimester or at delivery, in combination with the IgM predominance and lag in production of IgG in the primary immune response. In subsequent pregnancies, HDF/HDN has an earlier onset in gestation and is more severe, reflecting a more vigorous, anamnestic maternal immune response with rapid generation of IgG upon reexposure to incompatible fetal red cells. Nonimmune causes of hydrops fetalis include severe chronic anemia resulting from alpha thalassemia, cardiac disease, or intrauterine infection.

ABO incompatibility prevails as the most common cause of HDN, affecting about 0.7% to 2% of infants.[11] IgG ABO isoagglutinins occur without prior red cell exposure. High titers of IgG antibodies are more likely to occur in group O individuals than in group A or B individuals, and anti-A1 is more often associated with hemolysis than anti-B. Consequently, first-born infants may demonstrate ABO HDN, and those born to group O mothers, especially type A infants, are preferentially affected. Group O mothers with ABO-incompatible infants account for 15% of all pregnancies, and ABO antibodies can be detected after birth in the majority of these cases with sensitive techniques. However, only 4% to 11% of infants with maternal ABO antibodies have clinical signs of hemolysis, and less than 1% develop severe disease.[11] Anemia caused by ABO HDN tends to be mild or moderate because hemolysis is mitigated by several factors, including weak ABO-antigen expression on the infant's red cells and the absorption of the antibodies by A and B antigens in plasma and by vascular endothelia. Compensatory hematopoietic activity may be evident with occasional, circulating, nucleated, red cells and erythropoietic progenitors, but spherocytes predominate in the peripheral smear of infants with ABO HDN. Despite the propensity for mild disease in ABO HDN, the potential exists for dangerous levels of unconjugated bilirubin to accumulate because of ongoing hemolysis. Unrecognized hyperbilirubinemia in infants resulted in 90 cases of kernicterus in a 17-year period, according to a 2001 Sentinel Event Alert from the Joint Commission on Accreditation of Healthcare Organizations.[12] Nonimmune causes of neonatal hemolysis and unconjugated hyperbilirubinemia include infections and inherited red cell disorders, such as hemoglobinopathies, red cell enzyme deficiencies, or membrane defects.

Laboratory Diagnosis

All pregnant women should have their blood type (ABO/D) determined and should be screened for red cell alloantibodies at their first obstetric visit.[13] This testing will identify D-negative candidates for RhIG administration and those alloimmunized women who require additional monitoring for fetal anemia.[13] If a pregnant woman demonstrates a red cell alloantibody that has been implicated in HDF, the probability that the fetus inherited the blood group allele can be determined by evaluating expression of the red cell antigen by the biologic father. Paternity must be certain, however, to draw conclusions to guide management. If the father lacks the antigen, the infant is not at risk and no additional fetal testing or monitoring is necessary. If the red cell antigen in question is present on the father's red cells, molecular studies to determine the father's genotype are possible for many red cell antigens, including the complex *RHD* genetic locus as well as allele-specific assays for other Rh (Cc, Ee), Kell (K1/K2), Duffy (Fy^a/Fy^b), Kidd (Jk^a/Jk^b) loci.[14] If the father is homozygous for the implicated antigen, all his offspring will be at risk of HDF/HDN. If the father is heterozygous, his offspring have a 50% chance of inheriting the blood group antigen allele, and further prenatal diagnosis may be warranted.[15] Amniocentesis is the preferred method to obtain fetal DNA, as early as 15 weeks' gestation, and will determine the fetal red cell genotype.[15] Techniques to isolate fetal DNA from maternal blood are not yet sufficiently reliable or accurate for use in routine clinical practice.[2]

Pregnancies at risk for HDF should be monitored by serial maternal antibody titers, Doppler ultrasound, and amniocentesis or fetal blood sampling (percutaneous umbilical blood sampling).[3,15,16] The critical titer of maternal antibody is defined as the titer associated with a significant risk of severe HDF, requiring aggressive intervention in utero, and is often 16 (range 8 to 32) for anti-D. A lower critical threshold has been recommended for anti-K1 because severe disease may occur at lower concentrations of anti-K1 than anti-D.[3] Conversely, higher thresholds have been proposed for other antibodies, such as anti-M, that are less likely to cause severe disease than anti-D or anti-K1.[3] For all red cell alloantibodies implicated in HDF, a fourfold increase in antibody titer is considered a significant change that warrants further diagnostic investigation by amniotic fluid analysis or fetal blood sampling.[15]

Doppler assessment of the peak velocity in the fetal middle cerebral artery accurately detects fetal anemia and is used to monitor alloimmunized pregnancies in conjunction with serial amniocentesis. Doppler ultrasound may supplant the need for this invasive testing in the future, especially for Kell-sensitized pregnancies.[3,15] Serial amniocentesis to measure bilirubin concentration (ΔOD_{450}) is an indirect measure of fetal hemolysis, and trends are tracked on the Liley curve or Queenan curve, depending on gestational age.[15,16] Amniotic fluid analysis may be unreliable when HDF is caused by anti-K1, because these antibodies not only cause hemolysis but also suppress erythropoiesis as reflected by falsely reassuring ΔOD_{450} values in the setting of profound fetal anemia. Fetal blood sampling to directly measure fetal hematologic parameters is generally undertaken for extremely high-risk pregnancies or after amniocentesis or Doppler ultrasound suggest the presence of severe or worsening fetal anemia. The risk of fetal death is about 1% with amniocentesis and 1% to 3% with fetal blood sampling.

Immunohematologic testing of infants born to women with potentially significant red cell alloantibodies should include ABO- and Rh-typing as well as a direct antiglobulin test (DAT) at birth.[13] If HDN is suspected on clinical grounds but the DAT and maternal antibody screen are negative, the possibility of incompatibility should be investigated by testing the mother's serum or an eluate prepared from the infant's red cells against the biologic father's red cells. A negative DAT does not rule out the possibility of immune-mediated hemolytic anemia and may reflect a low antigen density on fetal red cells or low avidity of the offending antibody under the reaction conditions.[1] HDN is unlikely to be caused by ABO incompatibility when the infant's DAT is negative, and other causes of hemolysis should be sought.[17]

The American Association of Blood Banks (AABB) does not recommend routine immunohematologic testing of infants born to women with negative antibody screens, except as warranted clinically or to determine the RhIG candidacy of Rh-negative mothers.[13] Regardless, many institutions continue to perform ABO/D typing and a DAT on all newborns; others selectively test infants born to group O mothers. The latter strategy, which is intended to identify infants at risk of developing ABO HDN, suffers from an extremely poor predictive value and the potential to miss cases of hemolysis resulting from other causes. All infants should be monitored for hyperbilirubinemia in the first weeks of life, and serologic testing of infants should be prompted by the development of neonatal jaundice, unexplained anemia with reticulocytosis, or both.[13]

Prevention

Alloimmunization to the D antigen in D-negative women may be prevented by administering RhIG at 28 weeks' gestation and within 72 hours of delivery or other potentially sensitizing events (see Table 16).[4] If the 72-hour interval is exceeded, RhIG should

Table 16. RhIG to Prevent D Alloimmunization in Pregnancy*

Pregnancy and Delivery
   Antenatal: At 28 weeks[†]
   Postpartum: After delivery of D-positive infant, with additional doses as needed for FMH greater than 30 mL whole blood (15 mL D-positive red cells) (see Table 17)
Abortion
   Induced abortion
   Spontaneous abortion
   Threatened abortion
   Second- or third-trimester antenatal bleeding
Ectopic pregnancy
Amniocentesis
Cordocentesis
Chorionic villous sampling
External cephalic version
Abdominal trauma

---

*RhIG administration (300 µg) should be administered to D-negative women without anti-D within 72 hours of delivery, abortion, or event. A standard dose (300 µg) should be administered for all indications, although in early abortion or potentially sensitizing events, a smaller dose (50 µg) is acceptable in the first trimester.[4] Many blood banks and pharmacies, however, do not dispense the smaller dose vials.
[†]Unless the biologic father of the infant is known to be D negative.
RhIG = Rh Immune Globulin; FMH = fetomaternal hemorrhage.

be administered as soon as the oversight is realized because prophylaxis has been shown to be effective up to 13 days, and possibly as late as 28 days, following exposure to D-positive red cells.[4] Women who possess the weak D phenotype demonstrate qualitative or quantitative differences in D-antigen expression compared to D-positive individuals. Alloimmunization to the D antigen and HDF/HDN due to anti-D is rare among weak D females. Consequently, the AABB does not require testing for weak D in pregnancy, and current recommendations from the American College of Obstetricians and Gynecologists (ACOG) advise against administering RhIG to women with known weak D phenotypes.[4,13]

The AABB endorses routine screening for FMH after a D-negative woman delivers a D-positive infant, to identify bleeding in excess of 15 mL red cells (30 mL whole blood) requiring administration of additional postpartum RhIG.[1,13] FMH of this magnitude, detected in less than 1% of pregnancies, is more likely following Cesarean sections or operative vaginal deliveries but can occur following uncomplicated vaginal deliveries as well.[18] The calculation of the dose of RhIG for a large-volume FMH is illustrated in Table 17.[1] Because multiple intramuscular injections of RhIG may cause significant discomfort and no more

Table 17. RHIG Dose Following FMH[1(p511)]

% Fetal Cells*	Vials† of RhIG to Inject	Dose	
		In μg	In IU
0.3-0.8	2	600	3000
0.9-1.4	3	900	4500
1.5-2.0	4	1200	6000
2.1-2.5	5	1500	7500

*Based on Kleihauer-Betke acid elution test.
†1 Vial of 300 μg (1500 IU) is needed for each 15 mL of fetal red cells or 30 mL of fetal whole blood.

Sample calculation

The number of 300 μg (1500 IU) vials of RhIG needed for a 1.5% FMH (Kleihauer-Betke acid elution), assuming a maternal blood volume of 5000 mL (75 mL/kg):

$$[(0.015)(5000 \text{ mL})] \div 30 \text{ mL fetal whole blood/vial RhIG} = 2.5 \text{ vials}$$

The calculated number of vials (2.5) is then rounded off according to standard convention to 3.0. One additional vial is added as a precaution, so that 4 vials (total dose 1200 μg/6000 IU) RhIG should be administered.

than 5 vials of RhIG (1500 µg) should be administered by this route at one time, the intravenous preparation of RhIG (eg, WinRho, Cangene Corporation, Winnipeg, Manitoba, Canada) can be used for massive FMH, as indicated in the package insert.

Treatment

Prenatal monitoring of maternal antibody titers, Doppler ultrasounds, and amniotic fluid studies may indicate the need for fetal blood sampling and intrauterine transfusion. Intrauterine red cell transfusion is generally undertaken when the fetal hematocrit decreases below 25% to 30% and is usually not performed until after 20 weeks' gestation.[15] Considerations for selection of red cell units for intrauterine transfusion are given in Table 18.[1,16,19] The volume required depends on the transfusion technique (eg, intraperitoneal vs intravascular) and approximation of fetal weight.[1] An average intravascular transfusion is 50 mL/kg nonhydropic fetal weight, transfused in 10-mL aliquots over 1 to 2 minutes. Intrauterine transfusions are usually given as straight transfusions rather than exchange transfusions, given the technical complexity of the latter. The goal of transfusion is to keep the fetal hematocrit above 25% to 40%; (50% is often the target) but this endpoint should not be exceeded more than a fourfold increase in hematocrit to avoid unfavorable viscosity changes in profoundly anemic fetuses.[15] Repeat transfusions are planned taking into account the approximate 1% decline per day in hematocrit following intravascular transfusion. Brisk hemolysis of fetal red cells with severe disease often necessitates a shorter interval between the first and second transfusions (7 to 14 days) compared with subsequent transfusions (21 to 28 days).[15] Intrauterine transfusions generally are not given after 35 weeks, with delivery anticipated at 37 to 38 weeks.

After birth, the therapeutic approach to anemia and jaundice depends on the gestational age at delivery, birthweight, severity of disease, and concomitant illness.[20] Intrauterine transfusion often obviates the need for exchange transfusion in the neonatal period. Phototherapy is the first line of treatment for neonatal jaundice and may avert exchange transfusion. Exchange transfusion is usually needed, however, when phototherapy fails to ade-

Table 18. Selection of Red Cell Units for HDF/HDN[1,15,19]

Fetal Transfusion	Neonatal Transfusions	
	Exchange Transfusion	Small-Volume Transfusion
Group O, D-negative red cells lacking the implicated red cell antigen	• Group O, D-negative red cells lacking the implicated red cell antigen – OR – • ABO/Rh type-specific, lacking the implicated red cell antigen	• Group O, D-negative red cells lacking the implicated red cell antigen – OR – • ABO/Rh type-specific, lacking the implicated red cell antigen
Compatible with maternal serum	Compatible with maternal serum	Compatible with maternal serum
CPDA unit preferred (Hct, 75-85%) or AS units with supernatant removed (Hct, 75-85%)	CPDA unit preferred Reconstitute red cells to final desired hematocrit (40-50%) with AB-negative or compatible FFP	CPDA or AS units
Washed*	< 5- to 7-day-old units or washed if older	No requirement for washing or freshness
CMV reduced risk	CMV reduced risk	See Special Products
Gamma irradiated [25 Gy]	Gamma irradiated [25 Gy]	See Special Products
HbS negative	HbS negative	HbS negative

Table 18. Selection of Red Cell Units for HDF/HDN[1,15,19] (continued)

Fetal Transfusion	Neonatal Transfusions	
	Exchange Transfusion	Small-Volume Transfusion
Volume to transfuse (unit Hct, 75-85%)	Two-blood-volume exchange:	Up to 20 mL/kg
• Intraperitoneal transfusion: [(gestational age in weeks − 20) × 10 mL]	Term infants: 2 × 85 mL/kg (160 mL/kg)	10-15 mL/kg expected to give increment of 3 g/dL Hb/ 10% Hct if donor unit Hct is 75% or greater.[†]
• Intravascular transfusion: Blood volume (mL) = ultrasound fetal weight (g) × 0.14. Volume to administer depends on desired target Hct, which is between 25% and 50% depending on the pretransfusion value.[†]	Preterm infants: 2 × 100 mL/kg (200 mL/kg)	
	A two-blood-volume exchange removes 85% of red cells and 25-45% of serum bilirubin.	
Transfusion volumes generally range between 30 mL to 100 mL.	Transfused volume may be adjusted to achieve a higher posttransfusion hematocrit depending on clinical condition of infant.[†]	

*Some blood banks use washed red cell units to minimize exposure to incompatible plasma, additives, and potassium that accumulate with storage. Alternative strategies include fresh (<7- to 10-day-old) units or volume reduction.
[†]To calculate volume required to achieve desired increment in hematocrit:

$$\text{Volume to transfuse (mL)} = \text{Total blood volume (mL)} \times \frac{\text{Desired HCT} - \text{Pretransfusion Hct}}{\text{Donor unit Hct}}$$

quately decrease bilirubin concentration or when the initial serum bilirubin places the infant at high risk of kernicterus. Infants with jaundice caused by immune-mediated hemolysis are considered at greater risk of bilirubin encephalopathy than infants with "physiologic" jaundice at any given serum unconjugated bilirubin concentration. Factors potentiating bilirubin toxicity in the setting of hemolytic disease include acid-base disturbances, asphyxia, free heme groups, and other byproducts of hemolysis or drugs that displace bilirubin from albumin and other plasma-binding protein.

Published guidance on specific indications for exchange transfusion for HDN, however, is often based on older studies, which were performed before the development of effective phototherapy and prenatal intervention. Jaundice on the first day of life is always pathologic and requires individualized treatment decisions. Historically, criteria used for early exchange transfusion within 12 hours of birth include a cord bilirubin concentration exceeding 3 to 5 mg/dL for preterm infants, 5 to 7 mg/dL for term infants, or a rate of increase of 0.5 mg/dL/hour or greater.[20] Treatment decisions after the first 24 hours are guided by birthweight, bilirubin concentration, and the rate of its increase (>0.5 mg/dL/hour) (see Table 19). If exchange transfusion is performed, a transfusion volume approximately twice the infant's total blood volume is administered incrementally while aliquots of the infant's blood are removed over a period of 1 to 2 hours (see Table 18). A two-blood-volume exchange removes more than 85% of the infant's red cells but only about 25% to 45% of plasma bilirubin, which re-equilibrates between the intravascular and extravascular volume.[1] Consequently, infants may require more than one exchange transfusion before an acceptable bilirubin concentration is achieved. Considerations for selection and preparation of Red Blood Cell (RBC) units for neonatal exchange transfusion are given in Table 18.

Complications of exchange transfusion are uncommon, occurring in 7% of infants.[21] Routine treatment of anticipated citrate toxicity is controversial, but hypocalcemia may be monitored or prevented by administering intravenous calcium during the exchange transfusion (eg, 1 mL of 10% calcium gluconate halfway through the procedure); symptomatic hypocalcemia

Table 19. Treatment of HDF/HDN on Days 2 and 3 of Life*

Birthweight (g)	Phototherapy Threshold (Bilirubin, mg/dL)	Exchange Threshold (Bilirubin, mg/dL)
≥2500	15	18-20
2000-2499	10-13	15-17
1500-1999	7-8	13-15
1250-1499	Immediate or 5-6	12-13
<1250	Immediate or 4	9-12

*Jaundice on the first day of life is always pathologic and requires individualized treatment decisions.
Adapted from Peterec.[20]

should be treated appropriately. Calcium infusion may cause transient bradycardia.[21] Other possible complications of neonatal exchange transfusion include hypervolemia and volume overload, arrythmias resulting from citrate or hyperkalemia, air emboli, thrombosis of the umbilical vein, necrotizing enterocolitis, bleeding caused by dilutional coagulopathy or thrombocytopenia, catheter-related infection, and bacterial sepsis or viral transmission.[1]

Infants who responded to phototherapy alone or those who received intrauterine transfusion may not require exchange transfusion. However, they may need simple red cell transfusions during the first 1 to 3 months of life for late-onset anemia resulting from ongoing low-grade hemolysis or erythropoietic suppression. In general, the transfusion decision should be guided not only by the hemoglobin concentration but also by the reticulocyte count and, most important, by the infant's condition, particularly when the infant is lethargic, feeding poorly, or not thriving (see Blood Components). In case reports, erythropoietin has decreased the need for transfusion during the late hypoproliferative anemia associated with intrauterine transfusion and the alloantibody-mediated erythropoietic suppression seen with anti-K1 and anti-D.[22] Erythropoietin is given in a dose of 1200 to 1400 U/kg/week, either as 200/kg/day intravenously or 400 U/kg subcutaneously three times per week.[23] Additional study is needed to evaluate the effectiveness of erythropoietin in the clinical setting of HDN.

Neonatal Alloimmune Thrombocytopenia

Pathogenesis

Neonatal alloimmune thrombocytopenia (NAIT), the platelet equivalent of HDF/HDN, is caused by maternal alloimmunization against paternally inherited alleles, transplacental transfer of IgG-antibodies, and subsequent immune-mediated destruction of fetal platelets. NAIT, which is usually not recognized until after birth, often has its onset during gestation. The platelet antigen implicated in more than 90% of NAIT cases among those of European ancestry is human platelet antigen-1a (HPA-1a; formerly, Pl^{A1}); other implicated antigens include HPA-3a and HPA-3b.[1] In Asian populations, anti-HPA-1a virtually never occurs and anti-HPA-4b is the most important cause of NAIT. Those of African ethnicity are at greater risk for alloimmunization to HPA-2 (Ko) or HPA-5 (Br) than HPA-1a.[24] Incompatibility to HPA-1 arises in about 2% of pregnancies overall; approximately 5% to 10% of those women develop antiplatelet antibodies but only a fraction have affected infants. Genetic factors likely influence the risk of alloimmunization, and HPA-1a antibodies are detected more frequently among pregnant women who express HLA-DR52a or HLA-A1B8Dr3.[1] The incidence of NAIT is approximately 1 to 10 per 10,000 live births in the United States.[25]

Unlike HDF/HDN caused by anti-D or other red cell alloantibodies, NAIT often affects a woman's first pregnancy, with 40% to 60% of cases in primigravidae, even though platelet antibodies are not "naturally occurring" as are ABO IgG isohemagglutinins. The majority (85% to 90%) of subsequent pregnancies are affected by NAIT, and the risk to subsequent offspring reflects the probability of inheriting the offending paternal allele. If the father is heterozygous for HPA-1a, the recurrence rate is 50%; if the father is homozygous for HPA-1a, the recurrence rate approaches 100%.[25] NAIT is often more severe in subsequent pregnancies.

Clinical Features

Thrombocytopenia at birth occurs in 50% to 75% of cases of NAIT but in only 5% to 10% of cases of maternal idiopathic thrombocytopenic purpura (ITP).[25] The majority (80%) of newborn infants with NAIT present with petechiae, purpura, or overt mucocutaneous bleeding within the first hours of life. The risk of intracranial hemorrhage (ICH) among severely affected infants with NAIT (platelets <50,000/μL) is estimated as 10% to 20%, with one-quarter to one-half of these episodes occurring in utero; in contrast, only 1% to 2% of infants born to women with ITP are at risk for significant hemorrhage. The overall mortality rate associated with NAIT is estimated as 1% to 14%. Among those infants with ICH who survive, more than 25% have residual neurologic impairment. Otherwise, NAIT is self-limiting because the maternal antibody is cleared from the infant's circulation, and platelet counts generally recover within 1 to 3 weeks.

HPA-1a antibodies are the most common cause of severe NAIT. Antibodies to HPA-5a generally cause less severe disease with mild thrombocytopenia and few, if any, hemorrhagic symptoms but have been implicated in cases of intracranial hemorrhage and death.[26] NAIT caused by anti-HPA-3a is similar in severity to disease caused by anti-HPA-1a.[26] Factors affecting the severity of disease in NAIT include the density of the target antigen expression on fetal platelets and the ability of the antibody to destroy or impair the function of fetal platelets. Unlike HDN caused by anti-D, NAIT cannot be monitored by following maternal antibody concentration because the titers do not reliably predict the risk to the fetus.

Laboratory

Thrombocytopenia (<150,000/µL) is common in the neonatal intensive care unit, affecting 20% of hospitalized infants. Among the many causes of low platelets in newborn infants are intrauterine infection, placental insufficiency, neonatal sepsis, or drugs, in addition to immune thrombocytopenia. Platelet counts below 50,000/µL at birth, however, warrant an immediate investigation for NAIT. The mother's platelet count is normal in NAIT but usually low in maternal ITP. The laboratory diagnosis of NAIT is often made by demonstrating relevant incompatibility between the mother's plasma and biologic father's platelets. Confirmatory molecular typing methods that are based on the polymerase chain reaction (PCR) are available for HPA-1a and other platelet antigens; the corresponding antibodies in maternal or neonatal samples are detected in serologic assays performed by immunohematologic reference laboratories. HLA antibodies may be associated with thrombocytopenia in the newborn period but do not cause NAIT.

Routine antenatal screening for NAIT among primigravidae is possible but not performed in the United States. No signs prompt prenatal investigation in a first-affected pregnancy. The risk of NAIT occurring in subsequent pregnancies can be assessed by determining paternal or fetal platelet antigen expression, and fetal thrombocytopenia can be monitored if incompatibility is demonstrated. As with prenatal diagnosis of blood groups, platelet genotype or antigen expression can be determined following amniocentesis or fetal blood sampling by molecular or serologic techniques.

Treatment

If NAIT is recognized during pregnancy, high-dose intravenous immunoglobulin (1 g/kg/week) with or without dexamethasone given to the mother has been shown to maintain or improve platelet counts in approximately 50% to 80% of fetuses.[27] Serial fetal blood sampling may be initiated at 20 to 24 weeks' gestation to follow trends in the fetal platelet count and to treat severe thrombocytopenia with platelet transfusion, if necessary. Compatible platelets should be available for each procedure because of the risk of severe hemorrhage and fetal death. Empiric prenatal treatment of the mother with intravenous immunoglobulin (IVIG) is an alternative approach in at-risk pregnancies.

After birth, high-dose IVIG (eg, 400 mg/kg/day for 3 to 5 days) may increase the infant's platelet count within 24 to 48 hours and is usually well tolerated.[23] Platelet transfusions may be given prophylactically when a more immediate increase in the platelet count is desired; for example, to correct severe thrombocytopenia in stable (<25,000 to 50,000/µL) or unstable (<50,000 to 100,000/µL) newborn infants or to treat signs of overt hemorrhage despite higher platelet counts.[23] Considerations for the selection of platelets for NAIT are given in Table 20. Platelets that express the antigen implicated in NAIT may paradoxically produce an adequate rise in the platelet count, possibly by binding maternal alloantibodies to reduce their concentration. Consequently, platelets from the general blood bank inventory should

Table 20. Selection of Platelet Units for NAIT (Fetal or Neonatal Transfusion)

ABO/Rh compatible

- General blood bank inventory (antigen untested) platelet units may yield an acceptable response, and should be used if compatible platelets are not available
- Compatible (antigen-negative) platelets for optimal response, 10-15 mL/kg for 50,000 to 100,000/µL increment
- Minimize incompatible plasma (eg, volume reduction or washing) if maternal platelets are used

CMV reduced risk

Gamma irradiated (25 Gy)

- For intrauterine transfusion or infants at risk of GVHD (see Special Products) be transfused if compatible platelets are not available and there is an urgent need for transfusion. Compatible platelets may be collected either from the mother or from another donor whose platelets lack the corresponding antigen and whose plasma is compatible with the fetal red cells. If maternal platelets are used, the platelet-antibody-containing plasma should be minimized by volume reduction or washing. Maternal platelets must be irradiated.

Neonatal Alloimmune Neutropenia

Pathogenesis

Akin to HDF/HDN and NAIT, neonatal alloimmune neutropenia (NAN) is caused by maternal alloantibody-mediated destruction of fetal neutrophils, most commonly those expressing human neutrophil antigen-1a (HNA-1a), HNA-1b, or HNA-2a.[1,28] HLA (leukagglutinating) antibodies, found frequently in multiparous women, do not cause fetal or neonatal neutropenia, probably because they bind not only to white cells but also to other tissues and plasma proteins. Incompatibility to neutrophil antigens occurs in about 5% of pregnant women overall; about 40% of women who are homozygous for a neutrophil antigen deliver an incompatible infant.[28] As with HDF/HDN and NAIT, a small percentage of those women become alloimmunized in pregnancy, and only a subset of infants demonstrating maternal antineutrophil antibodies will develop neutropenia. Neutrophil antibodies were detected in 5% of women with incompatible infants; NAN occurs in less than 1 in 1000 newborn infants, with severe neutropenia affecting about 1 in 6000.[28] As with NAIT, about 40% of cases occur among first-born children.

Clinical Features

Neutropenia (<1000 to 2000 neutrophils/µL) is common among newborn infants in the intensive care unit, affecting as many as 8% of infants at some point during their hospitalization.[28] Although not specific for sepsis, neutropenia usually triggers immediate prophylactic treatment with parenteral antibiotics, even if bacterial cultures are negative, because of the high mortality rate of neonatal infections. Neutropenia in an otherwise asymptomatic infant may result from maternal alloimmune neutropenia, maternal autoimmune neutropenia, or other causes. Immune-mediated neutropenia caused by maternal antibodies is self-limiting and resolves within 2 to 4 weeks, but it may be severe and may last as long as 6 months.

Laboratory

The neutrophil counts of newborn infants exhibit wide variability and are generally higher in full-term infants than in preterm infants. Among full-term infants, the mean neutrophil count is 11,000/µL (6000 to 26,000/µL) at birth, with peak neutrophilia occurring at about 12 hours. By the end of the second week of life, mean neutrophil counts more closely approximate adult levels at 4500/µL (1000 to 9500/µL). Consequently, neutropenia is generally defined as less than 2000/µL in full-term newborn infants in the first 2 weeks of life and less than 1000/µL onward. Neutropenia occurs at birth in infants with NAN, but the maternal neutrophil count is normal. Confirmatory tests for granulocyte antibodies are performed in immunohematology reference laboratories.[1]

Treatment

Treatment of infants with neutropenia usually consists of antibiotics for presumed sepsis, followed by watchful waiting for signs of infection.[23] Severe neutropenia (ANC <500/µL) or prolonged neutropenia may be treated with recombinant granulocyte colony-stimulating growth factor (G-CSF, 5 µg/kg/day) for 2 to 3 days.[23,29] Prophylactic granulocyte transfusions are never indicated for isolated neutropenia; granulocyte transfusions are reserved for septic infants failing antibiotics and IVIG, with profound neutropenia and a diminished marrow neutrophil reserve (see Blood Components).[23]

Alloimmune Cytopenias Resulting from Blood Transfusion Therapy

Although newborn infants are susceptible to cytopenias caused by maternal antibodies, primary alloimmunization to red cell or platelet antigens with transfusion is extremely rare in the first months of life.[30] The practical consequences of a neonate's relatively unresponsive immune system, as well as the neonate's propensity to develop physiologic anemia and a susceptibility to iatrogenic anemia with frequent blood sampling, are different pretransfusion testing requirements for infants less than 4 months old (see Table 21).[1] Because any red cell IgG alloantibodies detected in the newborn infant are acquired from the mother during gestation, maternal plasma or serum may be used for pretransfusion testing instead of a sample from the infant. Repeat testing and crossmatching are not required during the hospitalization if red cells that lack the implicated antigens are transfused to the infant. Maternal IgG antibody persists in the infant's circulation for about 4 to 6 weeks, and standard pretransfusion testing protocols are required after 4 months.

Beyond the newborn period, pediatric patients may develop alloantibodies following blood component transfusion, and children with sickle cell disease (SCD) are historically at greatest risk of red cell alloimmunization. Alloimmunization to platelet antigens and refractoriness to platelet transfusion may be problematic in pediatric oncology patients or other children who are dependent on platelet transfusion. Transfusion therapy for actively alloimmunized children aims to provide blood components lacking the corresponding antigen. Adjunctive treatment strategies are directed at modulating the immune response of severely affected children.

Red Cell Alloimmunization in Sickle Cell Disease

Red cell alloimmunization among children with SCD is estimated to occur at frequencies ranging from 18% to 47%, compared with 5% to 11% in chronically transfused thalassemia patients and 0.2% to 2.6% in the general population.[31] The risk of red cell

Table 21. Special Considerations: Pretransfusion Testing in Pediatrics

Neonatal (<4 months old)	General	Sickle Cell Disease
Initial testing with sample from mother or infant: • ABO/D type [red cell (forward) group only]; Plasma typing (reverse group) not required • Antibody screen • Test for maternal IgG ABO isohemagglutinins, for type-specific transfusion only Repeat testing (ABO/D type, antibody screen): • Not required during hospitalization • Crossmatch is not required • Select antigen-negative units if maternal antibody present in initial screen	Initial testing: • ABO/D type • Antibody screen Repeat testing must be performed on a sample obtained within 3 days of the next scheduled transfusion, if the patient has been pregnant or transfused in the preceding 3 months • Crossmatch before every transfusion • Select antigen-negative units for history of clinically significant alloantibody	Initial testing: • ABO/D type • Extended red cell phenotype Rh (Cc,Ee) Kell, Kidd, Duffy, Lewis, and MNSs • Antibody screen Repeat testing, as for general patient population • Repeat antibody screen within 1-2 weeks after every transfusion is recommended if there will be prolonged intervals between transfusions • Select C-, E-, K1-matched units for all patients with sickle cell disease • Crossmatch before every transfusion • Select antigen-negative units for history of clinically significant alloantibody • Perform additional phenotype matching (eg, Duffy, Kidd) for those sickle cell patients with multiple alloantibodies, autoantibodies, or history of hemolytic transfusion reactions

alloimmunization increases with the number of red cell units transfused. However, children who receive transfusions before the age of 10 are less likely to become alloimmunized than adults despite exposure to more RBC units in their lifetime, possibly because of the induction of immune tolerance in those children.[30]

The primary cause of high red cell alloimmunization rates in children with SCD is the genetic disparity between the patient population and the general blood donor population. Many red cell antigens, such as C and E in the Rhesus blood group and K1 (Kell) are more commonly found in Caucasians than African-Americans.[1] Because African-Americans are disproportionately affected in SCD but underrepresented in the general blood donor population, almost two-thirds of the clinically significant alloantibodies found in chronically transfused sickle cell patients are directed against C, E, or K1.[31] Antibodies to Duffy, MNSs, and Kidd blood group antigens, primarily anti-Fy^a, -S, and -Jk^b, respectively, account for most of the remaining cases.

Complications of red cell alloimmunization include hemolytic transfusion reactions, autoantibody formation, and decreased availability of compatible RBC units. Prolonged intervals between transfusions predispose to delayed hemolytic transfusion reactions because the antibody titer may decrease so that it is no longer detectable in routine pretransfusion screening tests. Delayed hemolytic transfusion reactions occur 2 days to 2 weeks after re-exposure to the implicated antigen and are associated with mild hemolysis in most clinical settings. In patients with SCD, however, delayed hemolytic transfusion reactions are more common, occurring in 4% to 22% of patients, and may result in severe life-threatening anemia.[31] Hyperhemolysis or the hemolytic transfusion reaction syndrome in patients with SCD is characterized by the development of severe anemia after transfusion, with a decrease in a patient's hemoglobin concentration to less than the pretransfusion value.[32,33] Bystander hemolysis of autologous cells as well as transfused cells, suppressed erythropoiesis, and autoantibody formation may contribute to the profound posttransfusion anemia in those cases.[33] Autoantibodies affect 3% to 8% of patients with SCD, are most commonly detected in individuals demonstrating red cell alloantibodies, and may be clinically silent or associated with fatal posttransfusion hemolysis.[32]

Transfusion therapy of patients with SCD who have experienced such reactions, or have demonstrated multiple red cell alloantibodies and autoantibodies, must be individually tailored. The risk of additional red cell antibody formation and the possibility of fatal hemolytic transfusion reactions must be balanced against the potential benefits of red cell transfusion to alleviate acute complications and to prevent the chronic morbidity of SCD. In general, red cell transfusion should be avoided in patients who have experienced severe hemolytic transfusion reactions. These patients may benefit instead from pharmacologic therapy with steroids, IVIG, erythropoietin, or hydroxyurea.[32,34]

Prevention of Red Cell Alloimmunization in SCD

Standard blood bank practices are designed to prevent delayed hemolytic transfusion reactions and include accurate recordkeeping of prior red cell alloantibodies and avoidance of re-exposure to implicated red cell antigens for all future transfusions.[1] Further preventive measures for patients with SCD include obtaining an accurate patient history regarding previous transfusions at other institutions. Because red cell antibody concentrations wane following transfusion, screening for newly acquired alloantibodies 1 to 2 months after each transfusion has been recommended, but this precaution often is not practiced because it requires subsequent follow-up visits. Primary red cell alloimmunization may be prevented by avoiding medically unnecessary transfusions and by minimizing the potential for blood group antigen incompatibility between the blood donor and transfusion recipient. By prophylactically matching for C, E, and K1 blood group antigens, the alloimmunization rate among chronically transfused patients with SCD was reduced from 3% to 0.5% per unit, and hemolytic transfusion reactions were reduced by 90%.[35] Recent clinical practice guidelines propose that all patients with SCD should have their extended red cell antigen phenotype (ABO, Rh, Kell, Kidd, Duffy, Lewis, and MNSs blood group systems) determined before they start transfusion therapy; and they should receive ABO/Rh type-specific units that are phenotypically matched for C, E, and K1 and leukocyte reduced.[36] More extensive antigen matching is recommended for those patients who develop red cell alloantibodies (Table 21).[36,37]

Prophylactic red cell antigen matching for patients with SCD is not universally endorsed, however, and others advocate reserving this approach for patients with alloantibodies or those who have experienced hemolytic transfusion reactions. A more global strategy to increase African-American donor recruitment and to direct this blood to patients with SCD decreases the probability of antigenic mismatches, facilitates the identification of phenotypically matched units, and may further reduce the risk of alloimmunization.[31] Alloimmunization to blood group antigens in all other pediatric transfusion recipients can be managed by providing antigen-negative red cells after identifying the alloantibody, without the need for extensive pretransfusion phenotyping.

Simple vs Exchange Transfusion for SCD

Evidence-based clinical guidelines and consensus statements have outlined indications for transfusion in sickle cell disease, but the choice of simple vs exchange transfusion is often based on clinical judgment and available resources, with few clinical studies to guide decisions.[36] Both methods of red cell administration are effective in reducing the relative percentage of HbS containing red cells and in maintaining adequate hemoglobin concentrations. In preparation for surgery requiring general anesthesia, however, simple transfusion to increase hemoglobin to 10 g/dL was as effective as exchange transfusion in preventing perioperative complications in patients with sickle cell anemia.[38] The more aggressive exchange regimen was associated with a higher rate of red cell alloimmunization, resulting from increased blood usage in this group. Consequently, a conservative approach with the use of simple transfusion is recommended for prophylactic preoperative red cell transfusion in patients with SCD.[36-38] Simple transfusion can also be used for acute anemia, although increases in blood viscosity and impaired oxygen delivery will occur when the hematocrit is raised above 30% and HbS accounts for more than 25% of the patient's total hemoglobin. The benefit of exchange transfusion for acute sickle emergencies is the ability to rapidly decrease HbS concentration without simultaneously increasing the hematocrit or causing volume overload. No clinical studies have compared the efficacy of simple to exchange transfusion in these settings, so practice varies. In select clinical settings, the use of exchange transfusion offers advantages over simple transfusion and should be made available (Table 22).[36]

Chronic transfusion therapy to maintain the HbS below 30% of the total hemoglobin prevents first stroke in high-risk children with abnormal transcranial Doppler studies and prevents recurrent stroke in those with a history of infarctive stroke. The treatment goal for prevention of recurrent stroke may be relaxed to less than 50% HbS after several complication-free years, but treatment cannot be safely discontinued at any point.[31] An inevitable complication of long-term, simple transfusion is iron overload and the attendant cardiac, endocrine, and other organ-related toxicity. Although iron chelation therapy is effective, patient compliance is poor with the only currently available regimen—subcutaneous infusions of desferoximine over 8 to 12 hours daily. Oral iron chelators are not approved and demonstrate limited efficacy in clinical trials. Red cell exchange transfusion can prevent iron accumulation and may reverse iron overload in chronically transfused patients.[39] Disadvantages of red cell exchange include the need for more donor blood and increased donor exposures, as well as the insertion of a central venous catheter if peripheral access is limited. The potential risk of alloimmunization, however, is decreased with the use of phenotypically matched RBC units, and the potential benefit of delaying or preventing iron-induced organ damage may offset any residual risk of increased donor exposure. Finally, red cell exchange transfusion to prevent or treat complications in SCD requires an apheresis team experienced in pediatric applications.[39]

Alloimmune Thrombocytopenia

Platelet transfusions are frequently given to cancer patients with chemotherapy- or radiation-induced thrombocytopenia. Platelet antibodies have been reported historically in 18% to 50% of these patients.[1] Platelet antibodies are directed against Class I HLA or platelet-specific antigens, such as HPA-1a. The antibodies appear

Table 22. Transfusion in Sickle Cell Disease[36]

Accepted Indications and Preferred Transfusion Methods

Episodic or Acute	Chronic
Simple transfusion:	Exchange transfusion:
Management of severe anemia	Prevention of stroke in children with abnormal transcranial Doppler studies
Acute splenic sequestration	Prevention of stroke recurrence
Transient red cell aplasia	Chronic debilitating pain
Preparation for general anesthesia	Pulmonary hypertension
Exchange or simple transfusion:	Anemia associated with chronic renal failure
Sudden severe illness	
Acute chest syndrome	
Stroke	
Acute multiorgan failure	
Preparation for general anesthesia, if baseline hematocrit is too high for simple transfusion	

Controversial Indications

Priapism
Leg ulcers
Pregnancy
Preparation for infusion of contrast media
Management of "silent" cerebral infarct and/or neurocognitive damage

Inappropriate Indications and Contraindications

Chronic steady-state (asymptomatic) anemia
Uncomplicated pain episodes
Infection
Minor surgery that does not require general anesthesia
Aseptic necrosis of the hip or shoulder (unless indicated for surgery)
Uncomplicated pregnancies

as early as 10 days, but generally in 21 to 28 days, after primary exposure and 4 days after re-exposure to the antigen in patients previously sensitized through transfusion or pregnancy.[1] The risk of alloimmunization is related to the underlying disease as well as the immunosuppressive effects of treatment regimens. Alloantibody production was reduced during chemotherapy in adults with acute myeloid leukemia by reducing the leukocyte content of platelet components to below 5×10^6 per unit.[40] Limiting donor exposures by providing leukocyte-reduced apheresis platelet units did not offer additional benefit in preventing alloimmune-mediated platelet refractoriness over leukocyte-reduced pooled platelets derived from whole blood.[40]

Platelet refractoriness is clinically suspected when platelet transfusion fails to adequately increase the patient's platelet count. Immune destruction of transfused platelets must be distinguished from more common, consumptive causes of refractoriness, such as fever, infection, drugs, bleeding, splenomegaly, or disseminated intravascular coagulation. Under ideal conditions in pediatric practice, the expected platelet increment with 10 to 15 mL/kg of either whole-blood-derived or apheresis platelets is 50,000 to 100,000/μL. Optimal platelet responses in adults are 5000 to 10,000/μL per unit of whole-blood-derived platelets and 40,000 to 60,000/μL per unit of apheresis platelets. The response to platelet transfusion is more accurately evaluated by calculating the corrected platelet count increment (CCI) (Table 23).[1] Platelets may be destroyed rapidly by platelet antibodies, as evidenced by an unchanged or a minimally affected platelet count 10 to 60 minutes after the transfusion. In contrast, an adequate immediate response but poor 24-hour posttransfusion platelet count implicates increased platelet consumption by fever, drugs, or other nonimmune etiologies. Inadequate platelet doses often confound interpretation of posttransfusion platelet counts. After ensuring an appropriate dose of platelets and documenting at least two inadequate 10- to 60-minute posttransfusion platelet counts, the case should be referred to the blood bank/transfusion service for specialized patient testing and selection of compatible platelets.

Transfusion management of patients with alloimmune thrombocytopenia involves strategies to select HLA-matched or

Table 23. Evaluation of Response to Transfused Platelets[1(p347)]

Corrected count increment:

$$CCI = \frac{PI \times BSA \times 10^{11}}{n}$$

where BPI = platelet increment; BSA = body surface area; n = number of platelets transfused (expressed as 10^{11})

Example: If 4×10^{11} platelets are transfused to a patient whose body surface is 1.8 m² and the increase in platelet count is 25,000/µL, then:

$$CCI = \frac{25,000 \times 1.8 \times 10^{11}}{4 \times 10^{11}} = 11,250$$

Interpretation: This is an acceptable response to platelet transfusion. CCIs less than 5000 platelets/µL/m² within 1 hour of transfusion are consistent with immune refractoriness.

---

crossmatched platelets for transfusion or to avoid crossreactive HLA or platelet antigens.[1,41] The use of ABO-matched platelets provides optimal platelet recovery in this setting.[42,43] The patient's first-degree relatives are more likely than volunteer donors to share the patient's phenotype and may be a good source of compatible platelets. In some cases, however, immune-mediated thrombocytopenia cannot be managed with any transfusion strategy, and pharmacologic intervention directed at modulating the patient's immune response may be beneficial. IVIG (400 mg/kg for 5 days) improved 1-hour platelet recovery, but not 24-hour survival, of HLA-matched platelets transfused to alloimmunized, thrombocytopenic patients, suggesting a limited therapeutic effect at best.[44] Patients who are at risk of life-threatening hemorrhage and who demonstrate extreme refractoriness to HLA-matched or crossmatched platelet transfusion, however, have limited therapeutic options and justify a trial of IVIG.

Aminocaproic acid, an antifibrinolytic agent, has been used to control bleeding in adults with immune and nonimmune thrombocytopenia. However, unlike IVIG, aminocaproic acid may be associated with thrombosis or other unacceptable adverse events and should be used with caution in patients with cardiac, renal, or hepatic disease.[45] Rituximab, a monoclonal antibody that is directed against CD20 and that selectively depletes B cells, is a promising new agent for immunologic diseases, including immune-mediated thrombocytopenia, but experience in this clinical setting is limited to anecdotal case reports.[46] In extreme cases, therapeutic hemapheresis procedures have been used as a last resort to treat refractory alloimmune thrombocytopenia, but experience with this approach has been largely unfavorable.[1,47]

Platelet alloantibodies have been implicated in the rare complication of transfusion therapy, posttransfusion purpura (PTP), which usually affects multiparous women. One of the youngest patients reported to develop PTP, however, was a 16-year-old girl with no previous history of pregnancy.[48] PTP is characterized by the abrupt onset of severe thrombocytopenia ($<10,000/\mu L$) several days to weeks (average 9 days, range 1 to 24 days) after transfusion of platelets, red cells, or plasma.[1] Like the hyperhemolytic transfusion reactions in sickle cell patients, PTP destroys not only transfused platelets expressing the implicated antigen, which is often HPA-1a, but also the patient's own platelets, which lack the antigen. PTP is self-limiting and usually resolves completely within 3 weeks, but fatal intracranial bleeding occurs in 10% to 15% of patients. Treatment with IVIG (0.4 g/kg/day × 5-8 days) often results in rapid platelet recovery ($>100,000/\mu L$) within 3 to 5 days. Platelet transfusions should be avoided, but antigen-negative platelets may be beneficial for severe hemorrhagic complications.

Transfusion Support Following ABO-Incompatible Hematopoietic Transplantation

In contrast to blood transfusion and solid organ transplantation, hematopoietic (eg, marrow, peripheral blood) progenitor cell

Table 24. Transfusion Support for Patients Undergoing ABO-Mismatched Allogeneic HPC Transplantation[1(p556)]

			Phase I	Phase II				Phase III
Recipient	Donor	Mismatch Type	All Components	RBCs	First Choice Platelets	Next Choice Platelets*	FFP	All Components
A	O	Minor	Recipient	O	A	AB; B; O	A, AB	Donor
B	O	Minor	Recipient	O	B	AB; A; O	B, AB	Donor
AB	O	Minor	Recipient	O	AB	A; B; O	AB	Donor
AB	A	Minor	Recipient	A	AB	A; B; O	AB	Donor
AB	B	Minor	Recipient	B	AB	B; A; O	AB	Donor
O	A	Major	Recipient	O	A	AB; B; O	A, AB	Donor
O	B	Major	Recipient	O	B	AB; A; O	B, AB	Donor

Recipient			Donor	
O	AB	Major	Recipient	O	AB	Donor
A	AB	Major	Recipient	A	AB	Donor
B	AB	Major	Recipient	B	AB	Donor
A	B	Minor & major	Recipient	O	AB	Donor
B	A	Minor & major	Recipient	O	AB	Donor

RBCs	FFPs*	Platelets*
O	AB	A; B; O
A	AB	A; B; O
B	AB	B; A; O
O	AB	A; B; O
O	AB	B; A; O

*Platelet concentrates should be selected in the order presented.
Phase I = from the time when the patient/recipient is prepared for HPC transplantation.
Phase II = from the initiation of myeloablative therapy until:
 For RBC—DAT is negative and antidonor isohemagglutinins are no longer detectable (ie, the reverse typing is donor type)
 For FFPs—recipient's erythrocytes are no longer detectable (ie, the forward typing is consistent with donor's ABO group)
Phase III = after the forward and reverse type of the patient are consistent with donor's ABO group.
Beginning from Phase I, all cellular components should be irradiated and leukocyte reduced.

transplantation is not critically dependent on ABO compatibility between the donor and recipient. Major ABO incompatibility (eg, group A donor and group O recipient), however, may result in acute hemolysis of residual infused donor red cells, delayed red cell engraftment, and hemolysis at the time of donor red cell engraftment. Minor incompatibility (eg, group O donor and group A recipient) may be associated with immediate hemolysis of patient red cells from infused donor plasma or delayed red cell hemolysis caused by ABO isohemagglutinins produced by passenger lymphocytes. The hematopoietic product should be depleted of red cells or plasma, before infusion to reduce the possibility of the immediate complications of major or minor incompatibility, respectively. Following ABO-incompatible hematopoietic transplantation, blood component therapy is guided by the serologic findings during the transition from the recipient's blood type to the donor's blood type (Table 24).[1] Hemolysis caused by passenger lymphocyte-derived isohemagglutinins usually begins 7 to 10 days after transplantation and may persist for up to 2 weeks. If transfusion is needed during this period, group O red cells and plasma compatible with both the donor and the recipient should be used as long as the antibodies are demonstrated in the plasma.

References

1. Brecher ME, ed. Technical manual. 14th ed. Bethesda, MD: American Association of Blood Banks, 2002.
2. Bowman JM. Hemolytic disease of the newborn. In: Garratty G, ed. Immunobiology of transfusion medicine. New York: Marcel Dekker, 1994:553-95.
3. Moise KJ. Non-anti-D antibodies in red-cell alloimmunization. European J Obstet Gyn Reprod Biol 2000;92:75-81.

4. Prevention of RhD alloimmunization. ACOG Practice Bulletin Number 4. Washington, DC: American College of Obstetricians and Gynecologists, May 1999.
5. Chavez GF, Mulinare J, Edmonds LD. Epidemiology of Rh hemolytic disease of the newborn in the United States. JAMA 1991;265:3270-4.
6. Geifman-Holtzman O, Wojtowycz M, Kosmas E, Artal R. Female alloimmunization with antibodies known to cause hemolytic disease. Obstet Gynecol 1997;89:272-5.
7. Hoyert DL, Arias E, Smith BL, et al. Deaths: Final data for 1999. National vital statistics reports; vol. 49, no. 8. Hyattsville, MD: National Center for Health Statistics, 2001. [Available at www.cdc.gov/nchs.]
8. Vaughan JI, Manning M, Warwick RM, et al. Inhibition of erythroid progenitor cells by anti-K antibodies in fetal alloimmune anemia. N Engl J Med 1998;338:798-803.
9. Caine ME, Mueller-Heubach E. Kell sensitization in pregnancy. Am J Obstet Gynecol 1986;154:85-90.
10. Weinstein L, Taylor ES. Hemolytic disease of the neonate secondary to anti-Fy^a. Am J Obstet Gynecol 1975;121: 643-5.
11. Vengelen-Tyler V. The serologic investigation of hemolytic disease of the newborn caused by antibodies other than anti-D. In: Garratty G, ed. Hemolytic disease of the newborn. Arlington, VA: American Association of Blood Banks, 1984;156-7.
12. Joint Commission on Accreditation of Healthcare Organizations. Kernicterus threatens healthy newborns. Sentinel Event Alert 2001;18:1-4.
13. Judd WJ. Practice guidelines for prenatal and perinatal immunohematology, revisited. Transfusion 2001;41:1445-52.
14. Avent ND, Finning KM, Martin PG, Soothill PW. Prenatal determination of fetal blood group status. Vox Sang 2000; 78:155-62.
15. Moise KJ. Management of Rhesus alloimmunization in pregnancy. Obstet Gynecol 2002;100:600-11.

16. Management of isoimmunization in pregnancy. ACOG Educational Bulletin Number 227. Washington, DC: American College of Obstetricians and Gynecologists, August 1996.
17. Herschel M, Karrison T, Wen M, et al. Isoimmunization is unlikely to be the cause of hemolysis in ABO-incompatible but direct antigen test-negative neonates. Pediatrics 2002;110:127-30.
18. Ness PM, Baldwin ML, Niebyl JR. Clinical high-risk designation does not predict excess fetal-maternal hemorrhage. Am J Obstet Gynecol 1987;156:154-8.
19. Strauss RG. Data-driven blood banking practices for neonatal RBC transfusion. Transfusion 2000;40:1528-40.
20. Peterec SM. Management of neonatal Rh disease. Clin Perinat Hematol 1995;22:561-92.
21. Keenan WJ, Novak KK, Sutherland JM, et al. Morbidity and mortality associated with exchange transfusion. Pediatrics 1985:75:417-41.
22. Dhodapkar KM, Blei F. Treatment of hemolytic disease of the newborn caused by anti-Kell antibody with recombinant erythropoietin. J Pediatr Hematol Oncol 2001;23:69-70.
23. Calhoun DA, Christensen RD, Edstrom CS, et al. Consistent approaches to procedures and practices in neonatal hematology. Clinics in Perinatol 2000;27:733-53.
24. Kim HO, Jin Y, Kickler TS, et al. Gene frequencies of the five major human platelet antigens in African American, white, and Korean populations. Transfusion 1995;35:863-7.
25. Bussel JB, Zabusky M, Berkowitz R, McFarland JG. Fetal alloimmune thrombocytopenia. N Engl J Med 1997;337:22-6.
26. Glade-Bender J, McFarland JG, Kaplan C, et al. Anti-HPA-3a induces severe neonatal alloimmune thrombocytopenia. J Pediatr 2001;138:862-7.
27. Gaddipati S, Berkowitz RL, Lembet AA, et al. Initial fetal platelet counts predict the response to intravenous gammaglobulin therapy in fetuses that are affected by

PLA1 incompatibility. Am J Obstet Gynecol 2001;185: 976-80.
28. Zupanska B, Uhrynowska M, Guz K, et al. The risk of antibody formation against the HNA-1a and HNA-1b granulocyte antigens during pregnancy and its relation to neonatal neutropenia. Transfus Med 2001;11:377-82.
29. Maheshwari A, Christensen RD, Calhoun DA. Resistance to recombinant human granulocyte colony-stimulating factor in neonatal alloimmune neutropenia associated with anti-human neutrophil antigen-2a (NB1) antibodies. Pediatrics 2002;109:e64.
30. Strauss RG, Johnson K, Cress G, Cordle DG. Alloimmunization in preterm infants after repeated transfusions of WBC-reduced RBCs from the same donor. Transfusion 2000;40:1463-8.
31. Smith-Whitley K. Alloimmunization in patients with sickle cell disease. In: Herman JH, Manno CS, eds. Pediatric transfusion therapy. Bethesda, MD: AABB Press, 2002: 249-82.
32. Win N, Doughty H, Telfer P, et al. Hyperhemolytic transfusion reaction in sickle cell disease. Transfusion 2001; 41:323-8.
33. Petz LD, Calhoun L, Shulman IA, et al. The sickle cell haemolytic transfusion reaction syndrome. Transfusion 1997;37:382-92.
34. Ware RE, Zimmerman SA, Schultz WH. Hydroxyurea as an alternative to blood transfusions for the prevention of recurrent stroke in children with sickle cell disease. Blood 1999;94:3022-6.
35. Vichinsky EP, Luban NLC, Wright E, et al. Prospective RBC phenotype matching in a stroke-prevention trial in sickle cell anemia: A multicenter transfusion trial. Transfusion 2001;41:1086-92.
36. National Institutes of Health; National Heart, Lung, and Blood Institute. The management of sickle cell disease. 4th ed. NIH Publication No. 02-2117. Bethesda, MD: National Heart, Lung, and Blood Institute, 2002.
37. Vichinsky E. Consensus document for transfusion-related iron overload. Semin Hematol 2001;38:2-4.

38. Vichinsky EP, Haberkern CM, Newmayr L, et al. A comparison of conservative and aggressive transfusion regimens in the perioperative management of sickle cell disease. N Engl J Med 1995;333:206-13.
39. Kim HC, Dugan NP, Silber JH, et al. Erythrocytapheresis therapy to reduce iron overload in chronically transfused patients with sickle cell disease. Blood 1994; 83:1136-42.
40. The Trial to Reduce Alloimmunization to Platelets Study Group. Leukocyte reduction and ultraviolet B irradiation of platelets to prevent alloimmunization and refractoriness to platelet transfusions. N Engl J Med 1997;337: 1861-9.
41. Petz LD, Garratty G, Calhoun L, et al. Selecting donors of platelets for refractory patients on the basis of HLA specificity. Transfusion 2000;40:1446-56.
42. Ogasawara K, Ueki J, Takenaka M, Furhata K. Study on the expression of ABH antigens on platelets. Blood 1993; 82:993-9.
43. Jiménez TM, Patel SB, Pineda AA, et al. Factors that influence platelet recovery after transfusion: Resolving donor quality from ABO compatibility. Transfusion 2003;43: 328-34.
44. Kickler T, Braine HG, Piantadosi S, et al. A randomized, placebo-controlled trial of intravenous gammaglobulin in alloimmunized thrombocytopenic patients. Blood 1990; 75:313-16.
45. Bartholomew JR, Salgia R, Bell WR. Control of bleeding in patients with immune and nonimmune thrombocytopenia with aminocaproic acid. Arch Intern Med 1989;149: 1959-61.
46. Ratanatharathorn V, Carson E, Reynolds C, et al. Anti-CD20 chimeric monoclonal antibody treatment of refractory immune-mediated thrombocytopenia in a patient with chronic graft-versus-host disease. Ann Intern Med 2000; 133:275-9.
47. Grima KM. Therapeutic apheresis in hematological and oncological diseases. J Clin Apheresis 2000;15:28-52.

48. Chapman JF, Murphy MF, Berney SI, et al. Post-transfusion purpura associated with anti-Bak^a and anti-Pl^{A2} platelet antibodies and delayed hemolytic transfusion reactions. Vox Sang 1987;52:313-17.

HEMOSTATIC DISORDERS

Overview of Hemostasis

Normal hemostasis has three phases. First, blood vessels and cellular blood elements, primarily platelets, form the initial platelet plug at the site of endothelial disruption. Second, procoagulation proteins (clotting or coagulation factors) activate and produce a stable fibrin clot. Third, the fibrinolytic system and anticoagulant proteins limit clot formation to the sites of injury. Pathologic bleeding or thrombosis may result from derangements in any of these processes.

Platelet Function

Platelets form the initial plug at the site of endothelial disruption in the first phase of hemostasis. Activated platelets serve an important role in the procoagulant system by providing coagulation proteins and Ca^{++} during degranulation and a phospholipid surface on which coagulation factors assemble.

Platelet Function in Neonates

Bleeding times are shorter in healthy newborns and are longer in children than in adults.[1-3] Studies using platelet function analyzer 100 (PFA 100) assays (an in-vitro measure of bleeding time) have shown platelets of neonates to be both hyperresponsive and hyporesponsive depending on the sample type and test conditions.[4-6] The shorter bleeding time may primarily reflect the high levels of von Willebrand factor (vWF) and higher hematocrits in neonates, both of which independently augment platelet function and shorten bleeding time.[5-7]

Traditional platelet aggregation studies are difficult to interpret in neonates because of the lack of reference range values, but, in general, they show hyporesponsiveness to several aggregation agents.[5] Platelet aggregation in (mean age 9.3 years) pediatric patients is comparable to that in adults.[5]

Disorders of Platelet Function

Platelet function defects may be congenital or acquired. Congenital disorders include abnormalities of platelet granules or membrane receptors. Children with uremia and those undergoing procedures using extracorporeal circulation often have acquired dysfunction.

Platelet function defects are usually documented with platelet aggregation studies. Interpretation of results in neonates may be complicated, however, given the wide range of normal function in this population. The bleeding time is rarely ascertained in pediatric patients. Not only does the test cause scarring, but also the results may not be predictive of the presence of a bleeding disorder.[8,9] The closure time is an in-vitro bleeding time, performed by PFA 100. Closure time refers to the time required for a platelet aggregate to occlude the aperture of a collagen-coated membrane.[4,10] It is sensitive to platelet aggregation abnormalities (aspirin effect, Glanzmann's thrombasthenia) and von Willebrand disease (vWD). Many institutions have replaced bleeding time assays with closure time assays. Neither of those tests is superior to a detailed bleeding history. Abnormal closure time with an adequate platelet count should be followed by a platelet aggregation study, measurements of vWf, or both.

The most common hereditary bleeding disorder is vWD, which is transmitted as an autosomal dominant trait.[11] It may result from quantitative or qualitative abnormalities of vWF, a large multimeric molecule that binds, carries, and protects Factor

VIII in plasma. Platelet adhesion to subendothelial tissue requires vWF; therefore, platelet plug formation is deficient in patients with vWD, and the vWD induces a platelet function disorder. The vWD usually manifests itself as mucosal bleeding, but deep tissue bleeding can occur in severe cases. Because the level of vWF is increased in the first months of life, the diagnosis of type I vWD (all sizes of multimers present but at reduced levels) is difficult to make in the neonate.

Most forms of mild or moderate vWD can be treated with DDAVP.[12] DDAVP is contraindicated in individuals with the rare vWD type 2b variant and is not useful in type 3 variant where vWF is absent. DDAVP is usually given in doses of 0.3 µg/kg intravenously over 20 minutes. Most patients experience a twofold to threefold increase of vWF 30 to 60 minutes after infusion, and the effect persists for about 6 hours.[13] After several doses, the response is reduced as stores of vWF are depleted. Side effects include headache, facial flushing, fluid retention, and hyponatremia, which may be pronounced in children weighing less than 20 kilograms.

Factor VIII Preparations for Von Willebrand Disease

Patients who are unresponsive to DDAVP, those undergoing surgery, those with serious bleeding, or those who have vWD type 2b and type 3 variants require treatment with Factor VIII concentrates that contain vWF.[12] The vWF is co-purified with Factor VIII in plasma-derived Factor VIII concentrates, although preparations secondarily purified with monoclonal absorption contain very little residual vWF. Humate-P (Aventis Behring, King of Prussia, PA) is specifically approved by the Food and Drug Administration for treating von Willebrand disease in both children and adults. The vWF activity, expressed as ristocetin cofactor International Units (IU), is indicated on the label. The drug is usually given as a loading dose of about 40 IU/kg, with redosing every 8 to 12 hours. Hospitalized patients being treated for extended periods should be monitored by assaying levels after a steady state has been achieved (eg, after three or four doses) and every 1 to 2 days thereafter.

The Procoagulant System

The coagulation mechanism consists of a closely regulated series of reactions culminating in the formation of an insoluble protein gel called "fibrin." The initial platelet plug, which is woven with fibrin strands, stabilizes the clot. The system consists of enzymatic procoagulant proteins (Factors II, VII, IX, X, XI, and XII), non-enzymatic cofactors (Factors V and VIII), fibrinogen, and a fibrin-stabilizing enzyme, Factor XIII.

The exposure of tissue factor (TF) to blood initiates coagulation.[14] TF, present in the subendothelium, binds to circulating activated Factor VII (Factor VIIa) and the Factor VIIa-TF complex converts Factors X and IX to their active forms (Xa, IXa). Factor Xa with phospholipid and Factor Va convert Factor II (prothrombin) to thrombin. Thrombin, in turn, converts fibrinogen to fibrin, which is crosslinked and stabilized by Factor XIII. Thrombin amplifies the coagulation system by feedback activation of Factors XI, VIII, and V. This positive feedback sustains coagulation after the Factor VIIa-TF process is inhibited by the TF-pathway inhibitor.

Coagulation can also be initiated by the intrinsic pathway, which includes Factors XII, XI, prekallikrein, and kininogen. Contact factor deficiencies will prolong laboratory clotting tests but are usually not associated with abnormal hemostasis except for Factor XI deficiency, which can cause a moderate bleeding disorder.[15]

Screening tests of coagulation include: the prothrombin time (PT), which evaluates the integrity of Factors II, V, VII, and X, and fibrinogen; the activated partial thromboplastin time (aPTT), which evaluates the integrity of prekallikrein, kininogen, Factors II, VIII, IX, X, XI, and XII, and fibrinogen; the thrombin time (TT), which evaluates the fibrinogen-to-fibrin conversion step; and a quantitative fibrinogen assay.

The Procoagulant System in Neonates

The numerous differences in the procoagulant, inhibitor, and fibrinolytic components of the hemostatic system in neonates and young children, compared with adults, render these patients relatively hypocoagulable (see Table 25).[1,16-18] Most prominently, the levels of procoagulant factors are reduced. Except for fibrinogen, Factor VIII, Factor V, and vWF, the levels on day 1 of life in both premature and term neonates are only about half of those in adults.[1,3,16-19, 21,22] The PT is prolonged up to 2 seconds above the adult reference ranges, whereas the normal aPTT is 20 seconds or more above adult values in neonates with no clotting abnormalities other than the expected reduced factor levels. Progressive maturation occurs unless a coincident problem such as vitamin K deficiency or liver disease is present.[23] Adult levels are achieved by 6 months of age for some clotting factors but not until adolescence for others.[18] Premature neonates are somewhat more likely than term neonates to have achieved adult levels by age 6 months.[19]

Key inhibitor proteins (eg, protein C) and fibrinolytic proteins (notably antithrombin) are simultaneously reduced in the newborn, so that hemostatic balance is maintained and neither bleeding nor thromboses result unless the system is challenged or compromised.[11] Certainly serious bleeding complications occur in infancy, notably intraventricular hemorrhage (IVH) and periventricular hemorrhage in premature neonates. However, IVH does not appear to be a result of low levels of coagulation factors or any imbalance between the procoagulant and anticoagulant systems.[24-26] This finding is consistent with laboratory studies and clinical observations in adult patients with multiple-factor deficiencies (eg, liver disease), where factor levels above about 0.25 (25% of normal) are not associated with an increased bleeding risk.[27,28]

Empiric replacement of coagulation proteins with the transfusion of plasma is not recommended for healthy premature and term neonates despite the lower levels of procoagulants.[29] However, the reduced baseline levels do leave infants and young children with a reduced reserve if coincident processes lead to consumption (eg, disseminated intravascular coagulation, or DIC), increased requirements (eg, open-heart surgery), or dilution (eg,

Table 25. Approximate Reference Range Values for Selected Coagulation Screening Tests, and Coagulation, Anticoagulation, and Fibrinolytic Proteins*†

Test or Level	Preterm Infant, 30-36 GA, at Day 1	Preterm Infant, 30-36 GA, at Day 30	Term Infant, at Day 1	Children 6-10 Years	Adults
PT (sec)	10.6-16.2[16]	10.0-13.6[16]	10.1-15.9[16]	10-14[17]	10-14[17]
APTT (sec)	27.5-79.4[16]	26.9-62.5[16]	31.3-54.5[16]	26-36[18]	27-40[18]
Platelet count/μL	150,000-400,000[17]	150,000-400,000[17]	150,000-400,000[17]	150,000-400,000[17]	150,000-400,000[17]
Fibrinogen (g/dL)	1.5-3.25[17]	1.50-4.14[16]	1.67-3.99[1]	1.57-4.00[1]	1.56-4.00[1]
			1.75-3.5[17]	1.75-4.0[17]	1.75-4.0[17]
Bleeding time (min)				2.5-13[18]	1-7[18]
von Willebrand Factor	0.78-2.10[16]	0.66-2.16[16]	0.50-2.87[16]	0.44-1.44[18]	0.50-1.58[18]
Factor II (Prothrombin)	0.20-0.77[16]	0.36-0.95[16]	0.26-0.70[1]	0.67-1.07[1]	0.70-1.46[1]

Factor X	0.11-0.71[16]	0.20-0.92[16]	0.12-0.68[1]	0.55-1.01[1]	0.70-1.52[1]
Factor V	0.41-1.44[16]	0.48-1.56[16]	0.34-1.08[1]	0.63-1.16[1]	0.62-1.50[1]
Factor VII	0.21-1.13[16]	0.21-1.45[16]	0.28-1.04[1]	0.52-1.20[1]	0.67-1.43[1]
Factor VIII	0.50-2.13[16]	0.50-1.99[16]	0.50-1.78[1]	0.58-1.32[1]	0.50-1.49[1]
Factor IX	0.19-0.65[16]	0.13-0.80[16]	0.15-0.91[1]	0.63-0.89[1]	0.55-1.63[1]
Antithrombin	0.39-0.87[16]	0.48-1.08[16]	0.39-0.87[1]	0.90-1.31[1]	0.74-1.26[1]
α_2-Macro-globulin	0.95-1.83[16]	1.06-1.94[16]	0.95-1.83[1]	1.28-2.09[1]	0.52-1.20[1]
Protein C	0.17-0.53[5]	0.21-0.65[16]	0.17-0.53[1]	0.45-0.93[1]	0.64-1.28[1]
Protein S (total)	0.12-0.60[5]	0.33-0.93[16]	0.12-0.60[1]	0.41-1.14[1]	0.60-1.13[1]
Plasminogen	1.12-2.48[3]	1.09-2.53[16]	1.25-2.65[16]		2.48-4.24[16]

*Excerpted from Knofler, et al[1] Rand, et al[5] Andrew, et al[19] and Konkle, et al[20]
†All in units per mL unless otherwise indicated. Actual reference ranges vary between laboratories and for different reagents and assays. GA = gestational age.

total volume exchange transfusion) of functional clotting proteins (see Table 26).[30-34] In these settings, procoagulant deficiency may lead to an increased risk of bleeding and will require transfusion with blood components containing the deficient clotting proteins to prevent or treat hemorrhage.[35]

Abnormalities of the Procoagulant System

Both congenital and acquired disorders of coagulation occur in pediatric patients. Common congenital disorders include vWD and the hemophilias (single-factor deficiencies); common acquired disorders include liver disease and consumptive coagulopathy (multiple-factor deficiencies).

Table 26. Coincident Processes That Can Produce Clinically Significant Deficiencies of Coagulation Factors in Neonates

Consumption
- Disseminated intravascular coagulation
- Birth asphyxia[30]
- Sepsis
- Cardiopulmonary bypass
- Extracorporeal membrane oxygenation[31,32]
- Major surgery, including cardiac

Dilution
- Cardiopulmonary bypass[33]
- Extracorporeal membrane oxygenation[31-33]
- Total volume exchange transfusion[33]

Compromised production
- Vitamin K deficiency[23,34]
- Liver failure

Neonates and children with single-factor deficiencies should be treated with concentrates for the specific factor whenever available, because those factor concentrates may be recombinant protein preparations with no risk of disease transmission (eg, Factor VIII). The concentrates, derived from human plasma, have undergone specific treatment and processing to reduce or eliminate the risk of transmission of viral pathogens, in contrast to regular plasma components. This difference is of particular importance in pediatric patients who have a longer posttransfusion life expectancy during which long-term complications of transfusion-transmitted infections may develop. Additionally, factor concentrates can provide precise dosing at several times the number of units of coagulation protein per unit volume, compared with plasma for transfusion, thereby limiting the requisite total infusion volume.

Cryoprecipitated Antihemophilic Factor (AHF) is frequently used as a source of fibrinogen and for patients with Factor XIII deficiency. For deficiencies of Factors II, V, X, XI, protein C, and protein S, for which factor concentrates are not available, Fresh Frozen Plasma must be used for replacement therapy. Conditions associated with deficiencies of multiple coagulation proteins are also treated with Fresh Frozen Plasma (see Blood Components).

Single-Factor Deficiencies

Clotting factor concentrates are approved and available in the United States to treat hemophilia A (Factor VIII), hemophilia B (Factor IX), and hemophilia A with inhibitors (activated Factor VII and Factor IX complex). The vWF is co-purified with Factor VIII in the plasma-derived Factor VIII concentrates. The Food and Drug Administration has approved one preparation (Humate-P, Cangene Corporation, Winnipeg, Manitoba, Canada) for the treatment of vWD (Table 27).

Hemophilia A, Factor VIII Deficiency

Hemophilia A is an X-linked congenital bleeding disorder caused by Factor VIII deficiency. The vWF levels are normal. Patients

Table 27. Description of Clotting Factor Concentrates

Factor	Source	Preparation	Description	Comments
Factor VIII	Recombinant	Recombinate, Helixate, Kogenate FS, Bioclate, Refacto	Highly concentrated, no infectious risk	Product of choice for new patients
	Human plasma	Immunoaffinity or monoclonal antibody purification: Hemofil M, Monarc-M, Monoclate P	Ultrahigh purity, virus inactivated	
		Standard purification: Alphanate SD, Humate P, Koate HP, Koate DVI	High to intermediate purity, virus inactivated	
	Porcine plasma	Hyate C		For patients with high-titer inhibitors

Factor IX	Recombinant	Benefix	Highly concentrated, no infectious risk	Product of choice for new patients
	Human plasma	Single factor concentrates: AlphaNine SD, Mononine	High purity, virus inactivated	
		Prothrombin complex: FEIBA VH, Autoplex T, Konyne 80, Proplex T	Low to intermediate purity, virus inactivated	Thrombotic risk
Factor VIIa	Recombinant	NovoSeven	Highly concentrated, no infectious risk	Approved for hemophilia A and B with inhibitors; expanding off-label usage
von Willebrand factor	Human plasma	Standard purification preparations of Factor VIII: Humate-P, Alphanate SD, Koate HP, Koate DVI	High to intermediate purity, virus inactivated	Humate-P licensed for von Willebrand disease

with Factor VIII levels above 5% are considered to have mild hemophilia, and bleeding episodes usually occur only after significant trauma. Patients with moderate hemophilia have Factor VIII levels of 1% to 5% and may have excessive bleeding with minimal trauma or after surgery. Patients with severe hemophilia, with Factor VIII levels less than 1%, are at risk for spontaneous hemorrhage.

Mild or moderate hemophilia A can be treated with DDAVP, whereas severe disease requires the infusion of Factor VIII concentrates. Recombinant Factor VIII is the preparation of choice for treating young and newly diagnosed patients. The following formula is used to calculate initial doses to achieve levels of 30% to 100% (depending on the location of the bleeding or its consequence if bleeding were to occur) (Table 28)[36,37]:

$$\text{Desired units of Factor VIII} = \frac{PV \times [\text{desired level (\%)} - \text{initial level (\%)}]}{100}$$

Table 28. Desired Level of Clotting Factor in the Management of Bleeding in Hemophilia A and B*

Condition	Example	Target Factor Activity Level
Minor hemorrhage or minor risk if bleeding occurs	Early joint or muscle bleeding, hematuria, mild trauma	20-30%
Major hemorrhage or major risk if bleeding occurs	Extensive joint or muscle bleeding	40-50%
Life-threatening hemorrhage	Intracranial bleeding, surgery, gastrointestinal bleeding, head trauma	80-100%
Dental extraction		40-50%

*Association of Hemophilia Clinical Directors of Canada,[36] Lusher, et al.[37]

where PV (Plasma Volume, mL) = (1 − hematocrit) × 70 mL/kg × body weight (kg).

An alternative method of calculation is that each unit of Factor VIII infused per kilogram of body weight yields a 2% rise in the plasma Factor VIII level (ie, 0.02 IU/mL).[37]

Once a loading dose of Factor VIII preparation is given, subsequent dosing at 50% of the loading dose is usually given by intravenous bolus infusion every 8 to 12 hours. An alternative method of administration is continuous infusion.[38] Continuous infusion allows titration of the dose so that blood levels are predictable. Because very high peak levels are not needed to ensure adequate trough levels, the total amount of factor required to achieve a given degree of coverage is lowered. Drawbacks include the need for an infusion catheter and the use of the reconstituted product beyond the manufacturer's recommended limits, which may have implications both for risk of bacterial contamination and for factor activity.[38] The duration of treatment depends on the patient's response and the severity of bleeding. Hospitalized patients who require repeated doses or infusions should be monitored with Factor VIII levels to ensure adequate replacement. The level should be measured once a steady state has been established (eg, after the initial three or four doses) and then daily once or twice thereafter to confirm that minimum levels remain above the desired threshold.

Hemophilia B, Factor IX Deficiency

Hemophilia B is a congenital bleeding disorder resulting from Factor IX deficiency. The clinical manifestations are identical to those of hemophilia A.

Recombinant Factor IX is the product of choice for new patients with hemophilia B. Dosing is similar to that for Factor VIII (Table 28)[36,37] except that the loading dose has to be doubled to achieve any given target level of activity. The in-vivo recovery of Factor IX is only about 50% because of extravascular distribution. The dose is calculated as follows:

$$\text{Desired units of Factor IX} = \frac{PV \times [\text{desired level (\%)} - \text{initial level (\%)}]}{100} \times 2$$

where PV (Plasma Volume, mL) = (1 − hematocrit) × 70 mL/kg × body weight (kg).

Alternatively, each unit of Factor IX infused per kilogram of body weight yields a 1% rise in the plasma Factor IX level.

Once a loading dose of Factor IX is given, subsequent dosing at 50% of the loading dose is usually given by intravenous bolus infusion every 18 to 24 hours. Recent reports suggest that Factor IX, like Factor VIII, can be administered successfully by continuous infusion.[38]

Activated Factor VII

Recombinant Factor VIIa concentrates are approved for the treatment of patients with hemophilia A or hemophilia B and factor inhibitors. The exact mechanism of action of recombinant Factor VIIa is not fully known, but it probably works by enhancing thrombin generation through direct activation of Factor X.[39] For the intended and approved applications, Factor VIIa concentrates have been shown to be highly effective in both children and adults.[39-41] Dosing is not standardized and must be adjusted to the individual patient. Usually, several bolus doses separated by 2 to 3 hours are given to stop bleeding. Continuous infusion after a loading dose for surgery has been used successfully.[39]

This concentrate is increasingly being used in off-label settings for nonhemophilic patients who need a rapid, aggressive stimulus to clotting, most often in a surgical or trauma setting associated with uncontrollable hemorrhage. Recent case reports and small studies indicate a remarkable efficacy with apparently low risk of thrombotic complications (eg, DIC, myocardial infarction).[42] Factor VIIa has been reported to control pulmonary hemorrhage in very low birthweight neonates, life-threatening bleeding from a ruptured umbilical artery, bleeding following open-heart surgery in a child, and blood loss during orthotopic liver transplantation.[42-46] Nevertheless, these are all nonstandard applications of an expensive recombinant biologic only recently available. The risks of Factor VIIa are not fully characterized and doses are not standardized, which should limit use of this preparation to investigational settings.

The Anticoagulant and Fibrinolytic Systems

Regulation of normal hemostasis limits activities to the site of injury. Two main processes are involved: the natural anticoagulant system and the fibrinolytic system, which is responsible for the proteolytic dissolution of the fibrin clot.

In the anticoagulant system, antithrombin inhibits thrombin and other free coagulation factors. Alpha$_2$-macroglobulin, to a lesser degree than antithrombin, directly inhibits thrombin. Thrombin activates protein C, which, in the presence of protein S, inactivates Factor Va and Factor VIIIa.

Fibrinolysis is accomplished by the enzyme plasmin, which is formed by the action of endothelium-based activators on its circulating precursor, plasminogen. Plasmin binds to fibrin and breaks it down to soluble degradation products, leading to clot lysis. Unbound plasmin can degrade fibrinogen, Factor V, and Factor VIII. Plasmin, in turn, is regulated by plasminogen activator inhibitor (PAI) and alpha$_2$-antiplasmin.

An increased level of plasminogen activator, a deficiency of PAI, or a deficiency of alpha$_2$-antiplasmin may result in a bleeding tendency caused by hyperactive fibrinolysis. The laboratory hallmarks of an activated fibrinolytic system are shortened (<60 minutes) euglobulin clot lysis time, decrease in fibrinogen level, and accumulation of fibrin degradation products.

The Anticoagulation and Fibrinolytic Systems in Neonates

Plasma concentrations of antithrombin, protein C, and protein S are reduced, but levels of alpha$_2$-macroglobulin are increased in neonates. Alpha$_2$-macroglobulin remains elevated throughout childhood[2] (Table 25).

The fibrinolytic system of newborns is down-regulated. Plasminogen levels and the rate of plasmin generation are reduced in newborns, and levels of plasmin/plasminogen inhibitors are increased. The profile in children is similar to that in adults[11] (Table 25).

Disorders of the Anticoagulation and Fibrinolytic Systems

Primary disorders of fibrinolysis are rare and hard to differentiate from DIC. Antifibrinolytic therapy [eg, epsilon aminocaproic acid (Amicar, Amgen, Thousand Oaks, CA) or aprotinin] has been reported to be successful in the treatment of bleeding states associated with an activated fibrinolytic mechanism, such as cardiopulmonary bypass or liver transplantation. Anticoagulant factor concentrates are available for protein C and antithrombin.

Antithrombin Deficiency

Congenital deficiencies of antithrombin are associated with thrombotic disease. Antithrombin concentrates are used to treat patients with hereditary antithrombin deficiency, with plasma levels approximately 50% of normal, who have thrombosis or require prophylaxis before surgical or obstetric procedures.[47] Antithrombin concentrates are prepared from pooled human plasma and are heat-treated to reduce the risk of virus transmission.

Antithrombin concentrates have been studied as a replacement therapy in adult patients with septic shock complicated by DIC. In at least one European institution, neonates with sepsis are routinely supplemented with antithrombin when levels fall below 30%, although reports of the effectiveness of this intervention are limited.[48]

A recombinant antithrombin concentrate has been used successfully in small trials of patients with antithrombin deficiency who are undergoing surgery. This product is not yet available in the United States.[20]

Protein C Deficiency

Heterozygous protein C deficiency is associated with an increased risk of recurrent venous thrombosis. Homozygous deficiency results in a severe thrombotic disorder in the newborn period manifested as purpura fulminans and DIC. Newborns with purpura fulminans are usually treated with Fresh Frozen Plasma. Investigational (nonactivated) protein C concentrates are undergoing clinical evaluation.[49]

There have been anecdotal reports of use of nonactivated protein C concentrates to reduce mortality in patients with meningococcemia and neonates with sepsis.[48] A recently licensed recombinant activated protein C concentrate was shown to have modest efficacy in treating adult patients with severe sepsis and a high risk of mortality.[50,51] This preparation is not licensed for replacement therapy for protein C deficiency.

Other Hypercoagulability States

"Thrombophilia" is a term used to describe patients who develop venous or arterial thromboembolism spontaneously, at an early age, at an unusual site, or recurrently. Most patients have several acquired and genetic risk factors.[52] The most common manifestation is deep vein thrombosis of the leg or pulmonary embolism. Because neonates are ordinarily relatively hypocoagulable, a thrombotic event in this age group may be more likely to indicate a congenital thrombophilia.[53]

The most common inherited thrombophilic disorder is a mutation of Factor V. This mutation makes Factor V resistant to the inhibitory effect of activated protein C.[54] Between 1% and 8.5% of Caucasians are heterozygous for Factor V mutation, and the risk of venous thromboembolism is increased sevenfold. Cereberal venous sinus thrombosis has been reported in a 16-day-old premature neonate with heterozygous Factor V Leiden mutation, confirming that this condition may certainly manifest in the neonatal period.[55]

The prothrombin *G20210A* mutation is associated with elevated plasma prothrombin levels.[56] It is the second most frequent congenital risk factor for thrombosis. The gene is present in approximately 2% of Caucasians and in 6% of unselected patients with first thrombosis. Inheritance of this gene confers a nearly threefold risk for venous thromboembolism. Patients who are doubly heterozygous for Factor V Leiden and prothrombin gene mutations have a greater than 40-fold increased risk of thrombosis. The co-inheritance of these two mutations is also associated with a higher risk of recurrence of thrombosis.[57]

References

1. Andrew M. Developmental hemostasis: Relevance to hemostatic problems during childhood. Semin Thromb Hemost 1995;21:341-56.
2. Andrew M. The relevance of developmental hemostasis to hemorrhagic disorders in newborns. Semin Perinatol 1997;21:70-85.
3. Michelson AD. Platelet function in the newborn. Semin Thromb Hemost 1998;24:507-12.
4. Ortel TL, James AH, Thames EH, et al. Assessment of primary hemostasis by PFA-100 analysis in a tertiary care center. Thromb Haemost 2000;84:93-7.
5. Knofler R, Weissback G, Kuhlisch E. Platelet function tests in childhood. Measuring aggregation and release reaction in whole blood. Semin Thromb Hemost 1998;24:513- 21.
6. Rand ML, Carcao MD, Blanchette V. Use of the PFA-100 in the assessment of primary platelet-related hemostasis in a pediatric setting. Semin Thromb Hemost 1990;24:523-9.
7. Sola MC, del Vecchia A, Edwards TJ, et al. The relationship between hematocrit and bleeding time in very low birth weight infants during the first week of life. J Perinatol 2001;21:368-71.
8. Peterson P, Hayes TE, Arkin CF, et al. The preoperative bleeding time test lacks clinical benefit: College of American Pathologists' and American Society of Clinical Pathologists' position article. Arch Surg 1998;133:134-9.

9. Gewirtz AS, Miller ML, Keys TF. The clinical usefulness of the preoperative bleeding time. Arch Pathol Lab Med 1996;120:353-6.
10. Mammen EF, Comp PC, Gosselin R, et al. PFA-100 system: A new method for assessment of platelet dysfunction. Semin Thromb Hemost 1998;24:195-202.
11. Sadler JE, Gralnick HR. Commentary. A new classification for von Willebrand disease. Blood 1994;84:676-9.
12. Mannucci PM. How I treat patients with von Willebrand disease. Blood 2001;97:1915-16.
13. Hambleton J. Advances in the treatment of von Willebrand disease. Semin Hematol 2001;38(Suppl 9):7-10.
14. Dahlback B. Blood coagulation. Lancet 2000;355:1627-32.
15. Bolton-Maggs PH. Bleeding problems in factor XI deficient women. Haemophilia 1999;5:155-9.
16. Andrew M. The relevance of developmental hemostasis to hemorrhagic disorders of newborns. Semin Perinatol 1997;21:70-85.
17. Buchanan GR. Coagulation disorders in the neonate. Pediatr Clin North Am 1986;33:203-20.
18. Andrew M, Vegh P, Johnston M, et al. Maturation of the hemostatic system during childhood. Blood 1992;80:1998-2005.
19. Andrew M, Paes B, Milner R, et al. Development of the human coagulation system in the healthy premature infant. Blood 1988;72:1651-7.
20. Konkle BA, Bauer KA, Weinstein R, et al. Use of recombinant human antithrombin in patients with congenital antithrombin deficiency undergoing surgical procedures. Transfusion 2003;43:390-4.
21. Andrew M, Paes B, Milner R, et al. Development of the human coagulation system in the full-term infant. Blood 1987; 70:165-72.
22. Andrew M, Paes B, Johnson M. Development of the hemostatic system in the neonate and young infant. Am J Pediatr Hematol Oncol 1990;12:95-104.
23. Suzuki S, Iwata G, Sutor A. Vitamin K deficiency during the perinatal and infantile period. Semin Thromb Hemost 2001;27:93-8.

24. Andrew M, Vegh P, Caco C, et al. A randomized, controlled trial of platelet transfusions in thrombocytopenic premature infants. J Pediatr 1993;123:285-91.
25. Gleissner H, Jorch G, Avenarius S. Risk factors for intraventricular hemorrhage in a birth cohort of 3721 premature infants. J Perinat Med 2000;28:104-10.
26. Andrew M, Brook LA. Blood component therapy in neonatal hemostatic disorders. Transfus Med Rev 1995;9:231-50.
27. McVay PA, Toy PTCY. Lack of increased bleeding after liver biopsy in patients with mild hemostatic abnormalities. Am J Clin Pathol 1990;94:747-53.
28. McVay PA, Toy PTCY. Lack of increased bleeding after paracentesis and thoracentesis in patients with mild coagulation abnormalities. Transfusion 1991;31:164-71.
29. Roseff SD, Luban NLC, Manno CS. Guidelines for assessing appropriateness of pediatric transfusion. Transfusion 2002;42:1398-413.
30. Suzuki S, Morishita S. Hypercoagulability and DIC in high-risk infants. Semin Thromb Hemost 1998;24:463-6.
31. Zavadil DP, Stammers AH, Willet LD, et al. Hematological abnormalities in neonatal patients treated with extracorporeal membrane oxygenation (ECMO). J Extra Corp Tech 1998;30:83-90.
32. Arnold P, Jackson S, Wallis J, et al. Coagulation factor activity during neonatal extra-corporeal membrane oxygenation. Intensive Care Med 2001;27:1395-400.
33. Luban NLC. Massive transfusion in the neonates. Transfus Med Rev 1995;9:200-14.
34. Sutor AH, Von Kries R, Cornelissen EA, et al. Vitamin K deficient bleeding in infancy. ISTH Pediatric/Perinatal Subcommittee. International Society on Thrombosis and Haemostasis. Thromb Haemost 1999;81:456-61.
35. Roithmaier A, Arlettaz R, Bauer K, et al. Randomized controlled trial of Ringer solution versus serum for partial exchange transfusion in neonatal polycythaemia. Eur J Pediatr 1995;154:53-6.
36. Association of Hemophilia Clinical Directors of Canada. Hemophilia and von Willebrand's disease: Management. Can Med Assoc J 1995;153:147-57.

37. Lusher JM, et al. Medical and Scientific Advisory Council recommendations concerning the treatment of hemophilia and related bleeding disorders. New York: National Hemophilia Foundation, 1999.
38. Stachnik JM, Gabay MP. Continuous infusion of coagulation factor products. Ann Pharmacotherapy 2002;36:882-91.
39. Poon M-C. Use of recombinant factor VIIa in hereditary bleeding disorders. Curr Opin Hematol 2001;8:312-8.
40. Shapiro AD. Recombinant factor VIIa in the treatment of bleeding in hemophilic children with inhibitors. Semin Thromb Hemost 2000;26:413-19.
41. O'Connell N, McMahon C, Smith J, et al. Recombinant factor VIIa in the management of surgery and acute bleeding episodes in children with haemophilia and high responding inhibitors. Br J Haematol 2002;116:632-5.
42. Hendriks HG, Meijer K, deWolf JT, et al. Reduced transfusion requirements by recombinant factor VIIa in orthotopic liver transplantation: A pilot study. Transplantation 2001;71:402-5.
43. Chaunsumrit A, Nuntnarumit P, Okascharoen C, et al. The use of recombinant activated factor VIIa to control bleeding in a preterm infant undergoing exploratory laparotomy. Pediatrics 2002;110(1 Pt 1):169-71.
44. Aldouri M. The use of recombinant factor VIIa in controlling surgical bleeding in non-haemophiliac patients. Pathophysiol Haemost Thromb 2002;32(Suppl 1):41-6.
45. Jeffers L, Chalasani N, Balart L, et al. Safety and efficacy of recombinant factor VIIa in patients with liver disease undergoing laparoscopic liver biopsy. Gastroenterology 2002;123:118-26.
46. Olomu N, Kulkarni R, Manco-Johnson M. Treatment of severe pulmonary hemorrhage with activated recombinant factor VIII in very low birthweight infants. J Perinatol 2002;22:672-4.
47. Menache D, Grossman BJ, Jackson CM. Antithrombin III: Physiology, deficiency, and replacement therapy. Transfusion 1992;32:580-8.

48. Kreuz W, Veldmann A, Fischer D, et al. Neonatal sepsis: A challenge in hemostaseology. Semin Thromb Hemost 1999;25:531-5.
49. Dreyfus M, Magny JF, Bridey F, et al. Treatment of homozygous protein C deficiency and neonatal purpura fulminans with a purified protein C concentrate. N Engl J Med 1991;325:1565-8.
50. Bernard GR, Vincent J-L, Laterre P-F, et al. Efficacy and safety of recombinant activated protein C for severe sepsis. N Engl J Med 2001;344:699-709.
51. Ely EW, Laterre PF, Angus DC, et al. Drotrecogin alpha (activated) administration across clinically important subgroups of patients with severe sepsis. Crit Care Med 2003; 31:12-9.
52. Mannucci PM. The molecular basis of inherited thrombophilia. Vox Sang 2000;78(Suppl 2):39-45.
53. Abrantes M, Lacerda AF, Abreu CR, et al. Cerebral venous sinus thrombosis in a neonate due to factor V Leiden deficiency. Acta Paediatr 2002;91:243-5.
54. Dahlback B. Resistance to activated protein C caused by the factor V R506Q mutation is a common risk factor for venous thrombosis. Thromb Haemost 1997;78:483-8.
55. Ramenghi LA, Gill BJ, Tanner SF, et al. Cerebral venous thrombosis, intraventricular haemorrhage and white matter lesions in a preterm newborn with factor V (Leiden) mutation. Neuropediatrics 2002;33:97-9.
56. Poort SR, Rosendaal FR, Reitsma PH, Bertina RM. A common genetic variation in the 3-untranslated region of the prothrombin gene is associated with elevated prothrombin levels and an increase in venous thrombosis. Blood 1996;88:3698-703.
57. Margaglione M, D'Andrea G, Colaizzo D, et al. Coexistence of factor V Leiden and Factor II A20210 mutations and recurrent thromboembolism. Thromb Haemost 1999; 82:1583-7.

ADVERSE EFFECTS OF BLOOD TRANSFUSION

The decision to transfuse a pediatric or adult patient requires knowing and balancing the risks and the benefits. The beneficial effects can usually be appreciated on an immediate basis, whereas the adverse effects may be delayed or difficult to recognize in the presence of other concomitant factors that could obscure the clinical picture. Parents or legal guardians of pediatric patients should be advised of the risks, benefits, alternatives to, and consequences of refusal of transfusion. Documentation of the necessity for the transfusion and of informed consent is an essential aspect of transfusion therapy.

Acute Transfusion Reactions

Acute transfusion reactions occur during or within 24 hours following a transfusion. In most instances, the pathophysiology, diagnosis, and treatment of transfusion reactions in pediatric patients are based on knowledge gained about transfusion reactions in adult patients. Some of the more common acute transfusion reactions seen in children and adults, such as febrile or allergic reactions, are usually the result of an immunologically mediated event. These types of reactions are rarely reported in infants and usually are the result of passive antibodies.[1] Most life-threatening transfusion reactions occur early in the course of transfusion; however, acute reactions may occur after a transfusion has been completed.

As soon as an acute reaction occurs, it is essential to stop the transfusion immediately, keep the IV access open, verify

at the bedside that the correct unit was administered to the correct patient, treat acute symptoms (Table 29),[2] and follow hospital protocols for reporting the event and undertaking further investigation. If a reaction occurs during the course of a multiple-unit transfusion, the unit being transfused may not necessarily be the cause of the reaction.[3]

Acute Hemolytic Reactions

Hemolytic transfusion reactions (HTRs) are caused by the immune-mediated lysis of transfused red cells. Reactions may be either acute or delayed and may result in intravascular or extravascular hemolysis, depending on the nature of the antibody. An acute hemolytic transfusion reaction (AHTR) occurs when red cells are transfused to a recipient who already has a clinically significant preformed antibody to an antigen present on the transfused red cells, such as transfusion of group A red cells into a group O or a group B recipient. Patient misidentification typically occurs either when the blood specimen for compatibility testing is drawn or when a transfusion is administered. Misidentification is the most common cause of ABO-incompatible transfusion, resulting in acute hemolysis, and is the leading cause of death resulting from transfusion as reported to the Food and Drug Administration (FDA).[4] If the recipient's antibody fixes complement, as most often occurs with ABO-incompatible blood transfusions, an acute intravascular hemolytic transfusion reaction (AIHTR) results.[5] The anti-A and anti-B responsible are either IgM or complement-fixing IgG, both of which activate complement, resulting in the binding of the C5-9 component. Fixation of C5-9 results in the appearance of a pore in the red cell membrane that allows water to enter the cell, resulting in osmotic intravascular lysis.

Clinical symptoms associated with AIHTR are, in large part, attributable to the generated complement fragments, anaphylatoxins C3a and C5a, and to activation of the cytokine network, including the proinflammatory cytokines interleukin-1 (IL-1), IL-6, IL-8, and tumor necrosis factor-alpha (TNF-α). These biologic mediators produce fever, hypotension, and activation of white cells and the clotting cascade.[3,5] The binding of nitrous ox-

Table 29. Management of Acute Transfusion Reactions

Immediate steps for all reactions: 1) Stop transfusion; 2) Keep IV open with 0.9% NaCl; 3) Verify at bedside that the correct unit was administered to the correct patient; 4) Notify patient's physician and blood bank

When transfusion is terminated: 5) Send freshly collected blood and any necessary urine/blood samples to appropriate laboratory; 6) Send blood unit and administration set to blood bank

Type	Etiology	Presentation	Evaluation	Treatment and Prevention
Hemolytic (immune)	RBC incompatibility; ABO incompatibility usually caused by clerical error	<ul><li>Fever/chills</li><li>Hemoglobinemia/ hemoglobinuria</li><li>Anxiety</li><li>Nausea/vomiting</li><li>Pain</li><li>Hypotension</li><li>Renal failure with oliguria</li><li>DIC</li></ul>	<ul><li>Direct antiglobulin test (DAT)</li><li>Visual inspection for plasma Hb</li><li>Tests as indicated to determine RBC incompatibility</li><li>Tests to monitor hemolysis (Hb/Hct, haptoglobin, bilirubin, etc)</li></ul>	**Treatment:** Supportive treatment for hypotension and renal perfusion (maintain output >1 mL/kg/hour) may include<ul><li>IV crystalloid (ie, 10 to 20 mL/kg normal saline)</li><li>Furosemide[2] Neonate: 0.5 to 1 mg/kg/dose IV every 8 to 24 hours (max dose IV: 2 mg/kg). Premature infants will require less frequent dosing</li></ul>

(continued)

Table 29. Management of Acute Transfusion Reactions (continued)

Type	Etiology	Presentation	Evaluation	Treatment and Prevention
Hemolytic (immune) (continued)			• Tests to monitor renal function (BUN, creatinine) • Tests to monitor coagulation status (PT/PTT, platelet count, fibrinogen)	Children: 0.5 to 2 mg/kg/dose IV every 6 to 12 hours (max dose 6 mg/kg/dose) or continuous infusion 0.05 mg/kg/hour titrating dose to clinical effect • Low-dose dopamine (2 to 5 µg/kg/minute) Supportive treatment of DIC with active bleeding • Hemostatic components: platelets, FFP, cryoprecipitate **Prevention:** • Ensuring proper sample and recipient identification • Reviewing historical records • Providing antigen-negative units as appropriate

Reaction	Cause	Signs/Symptoms	Diagnosis	Treatment/Prevention
Hemolytic (non-immune)	Physical or chemical destruction of blood (thermal, drugs, solutions added)	Hemoglobinuria	• Plasma-free Hb • DAT (should be negative) • Visual inspection of unit for hemolysis	**Treatment:** • Hydrate **Prevention:** • Proper administration of blood components • Identify and eliminate cause
Fever/chill (nonhemolytic)	Antibody to donor leukocytes/plasma proteins Passive cytokine infusion	• Chills/rigors • Temperature rise (>1 C) not explained by condition • Headache • Nausea/vomiting Symptoms often occur near the end or after the completion of the transfusion	• Rule out hemolysis (DAT, inspection for plasma Hb) • Rule out bacterial contamination (culture patient and unit) Diagnosis of exclusion	**Treatment:** • Antipyretic, eg, acetaminophen 10 to 15 mg/kg/dose PO (avoid aspirin); for premedication, administer 30 to 60 minutes before transfusion **Prevention:** • Leukocyte-reduced component if recurrent • Premedicate with antipyretic, ie, acetaminophen 10 to 15 mg/kg/dose PO, 30 to 60 minutes before transfusion

(continued)

Table 29. Management of Acute Transfusion Reactions (continued)

Type	Etiology	Presentation	Evaluation	Treatment and Prevention
Allergic (mild)	Antibody to plasma protein	• Urticaria • Pruritis • Flushing	• Response to antihistamines	**Treatment:** • Antihistamine: children—diphenhydramine 1 to 1.5 mg/kg/dose PO/IV (administer 1 hour before transfusion for prevention of recurrent hives) • May restart unit if symptoms are resolved
(Moderate to severe)		• Respiratory distress • Wheezing • Laryngeal edema • Nausea/vomiting • Hypotension	• Rule out other etiologies for respiratory distress, eg, circulatory overload, TRALI, anaphylactic reaction • IgA levels • Anti-IgA	**Treatment:** (for anaphylaxis[2]) • Epinephrine 0.01 mL/kg (1:1000) SC (maximum 0.3 mL); can repeat in 15 minutes • In severe shock with severe hypotension, 0.1 mL/kg (1:10,000) IV, given slowly over 2 to 5 minutes • Diphenhydramine 1 mg/kg IV/IM/PO (maximum 50 mg); can repeat in 15 minutes

| (Moderate to severe) (continued) | Symptoms usually begin shortly after the start of transfusion. | • Albuterol nebulizer 0.05 to 0.15 mg/kg in 3 mL normal saline (estimate 2.5 mg <30 kg, 5.0 mg >30 kg)
• Methylprednisolone 1 to 2 mg/kg/dose IV

Prevention: (moderate reactions)
• Diphenhydramine 1 mg/kg/dose IV/PO 1 hour before transfusion
• Corticosteroids 2 to 6 hours before transfusion either: Methylprednisolone 1 mg/kg/dose IV
   Hydrocortisone 1 mg/kg/dose IV
   Prednisone 1 mg/kg/dose PO
• Autologous transfusion
• Washed components
• IgA-deficient component if appropriate |

(continued)

Table 29. Management of Acute Transfusion Reactions (continued)

Type	Etiology	Presentation	Evaluation	Treatment and Prevention
Circulatory overload	Too rapid or excessive blood transfusion or both	• Dyspnea • Cough • Rales • Rapid increase in systolic pressure • Headache • Cardiac arrhythmia	• Chest X-ray—bilateral infiltrates, may progress to complete "white out" • Rule out other etiologies for respiratory distress, eg, anaphylactic reaction, TRALI • Test donor/recipient for white-cell-related antibodies	**Treatment:** • Slow rate/stop transfusion • Upright position • Oxygen • Diuretics, ie, furosemide Neonates 0.5 to 1.0 mg/kg/dose every 8 to 24 hours (max IV dose 2 mg/kg/dose) Children 0.5 to 2.0 mg/kg/dose every 6 to 12 hours (max dose 6 mg/kg/dose) **Prevention:** • Transfuse blood slowly • Transfuse aliquots of blood

Transfusion-related acute lung injury (TRALI)	Passive infusion of donor HLA/leukocyte antibody through plasma-containing components; neutrophil-priming lipid mediator; recipient antibody to donor white cells—these mechanisms lead to microvascular injury in the lung	• Fever • Dyspnea • Hypoxemia, may be severe • Hypotension • Pulmonary edema • Normal pulmonary capillary wedge pressure	• Rule out hemolysis (visual inspection plasma Hb, DAT) • Culture recipient • Culture blood component • Rule out circulatory overload • Diagnosis of exclusion	**Treatment:** • Respiratory support may include oxygen, intubation/mechanical ventilation depending on severity of hypoxia • Blood pressure support (see above) **Prevention:** • If leukocyte antibody is present in recipient, use leukocyte-reduced blood components • If donor antibody is implicated, no special measures are needed for the affected recipient • May want to prevent the use of plasma-containing components from implicated donors in the future—inform blood donor center

(continued)

Table 29. Management of Acute Transfusion Reactions (continued)

Type	Etiology	Presentation	Evaluation	Treatment and Prevention
Bacterial contamination	Contaminated blood component (frequency is higher with platelet components than red cells)	• Rigors • Chills • Fever • Shock	• Blood cultures from patient • Culture transfused component	**Treatment:** • Support blood pressure (see above) • Administer appropriate broad spectrum antibiotics **Prevention:** • Careful attention to arm preparation for donor phlebotomy • Prevention of contamination during blood collection and storage
Hypothermia	Rapid infusion of cold blood	• Chills • Low temperature • Irregular heart rate • Possible cardiac arrest • Neonatal apnea		**Treatment:** • Slow infusion rate • Use blood warmer **Prevention:** • Transfusion with an approved blood warming device • Keep patient warm

| Hyperka-lemia (elevated serum potassium) | Hemolysis of red cells (immuno-logic/non-immunologic); massive/rapid infusion of blood with high potassium level | • Nausea/diarrhea
• Muscle weakness
• Cardiac arrhythmias
• Cardiac arrest | • Serum potassium (K^+) level
• Monitor EKG for peaked T waves, loss of P wave, widening QRS complex, ST depression, bradycardia/asystole | **Treatment:**
Depends on severity
• Cardiac monitor[2]
• Mild to moderate levels (K+ = 6.0 to 7.0 mEq/L), try to enhance excretion; Kayexalate resin 1 g/kg/dose every 2 to 6 hours
• Severe (K^+ >7.0 mEq/L), try to move K^+ into cell acutely:
Insulin 0.1 unit regular/kg with glucose 0.5 g/kg
Sodium bicarbonate 1-2 mEq/kg IV given over 5 to 10 minutes
• If EKG changes are present then urgent reversal of membrane effects is required: Calcium gluconate (10%) 100 mg/kg/dose (1 mL/kg/dose) over 3 to 5 minutes

Prevention:
Preventive measures for patients at risk for hyperkalemia:
• Fresh red cells
• Red cells with supernatant removed
• Washed red cells |

(continued)

Table 29. Management of Acute Transfusion Reactions (continued)

Type	Etiology	Presentation	Evaluation	Treatment and Prevention
Hypocalcemia (low ionized calcium)	Massive transfusion of citrated blood particularly in clinical setting of delayed citrate metabolism	Neonate • Jitteriness • Poor feeding • Apnea • Seizures • Arrhythmia Older children • Paresthesia • Tetany • Arrhythmia	• Ionized calcium level • Prolonged Q-T interval on EKG	**Treatment:** • Slow rate of transfusion • Prophylactic calcium during exchange transfusion is not routinely performed • Seizure activity associated with hypocalcemia should be treated: calcium should be infused IV slowly with constant monitoring of heart rate[2] Calcium gluconate (10%) 100 mg/kg/dose slowly **Prevention:** Monitor calcium during procedure and administer calcium as necessary

Hypoglyce-mia	Discontinuation of dextrose infusion during transfusion; rebound phenomena after exchange transfusion	• Jitteriness • Tremors • Seizure • Apnea/cyanosis	• Glucose level	**Treatment:** • If asymptomatic, maintenance glucose either PO (D5W) or IV 4 to 8 mg/kg/minute as required • If seizure activity associated with hypoglycemia: 5 to 10 mg/kg IV bolus (10% or 15% dextrose) followed by 8 to 10 mg/kg/minute IV drip as required[2] **Prevention:** Frequent glucose monitoring (30 to 60 minutes) during the transfusion; point of care glucose monitoring is optimal

[1]Holman et al.
[2]Siberry and Iannone. Doses and frequency may be altered depending on gestational ages as well as clinical condition of neonate/infant/child.
DIC = disseminated intravascular coagulation; IV = intravenous; IM = intramuscular; PO = by mouth; RBCs = red blood cells; SC = subcutaneous.

ide by free hemoglobin promotes renal vasoconstriction.[6] The combination of hypotension, renal vasoconstriction, and microthrombi formation in the renal vasculature contribute to the development of renal failure.

The severity of AIHTR depends on the rate and amount of blood transfused, as well as the clinical condition of the patient. Generally, the more incompatible blood given and the faster the infusion rate, the more severe the reaction.[3] If an AIHTR is suspected, additional Red Blood Cell (RBC) units should not be administered until the cause has been identified and corrected. In the absence of a red cell incompatibility, the search for a non-immunologic etiology for hemolysis should be initiated (see below).

Most AHTRs cause intravascular hemolysis; however, if the antibody implicated does not fix complement, or fixes only C3, the resulting reaction will be an acute extravascular hemolytic transfusion reaction (AEHTR). These reactions usually are not associated with the severe clinical symptoms seen with an AIHTR because there is less generation of the biologic response modifiers.[5] AEHTRs typically present with fever and are further characterized by a new positive direct antiglobulin test (DAT) resulting from antibody binding to the transfused incompatible red cells and a decreasing hematocrit without any overt signs of bleeding.[3]

Infants under 4 months of age generally have not yet developed anti-A and anti-B red cell antibodies or antibodies to other red cell antigens (alloantibodies)[1] and are not usually susceptible to these reactions. Maternal clinically significant IgG antibodies, however, can cross the placenta and in low concentrations may cause hemolysis of transfused red cells. Accordingly, the antibodies must be respected when the decision is made to transfuse. Many centers transfuse only group O red cells to neonates to avoid the possibility of ABO incompatibility. However, the use of type-specific blood is acceptable with additional appropriate compatibility testing. The passive infusion of incompatible isohemagglutinins from plasma or plasma-containing components—rarely from intravenous immune globulin (IVIG)—may cause severe hemolytic reactions. Although this reaction occurs more frequently with anti-A, acute intravascular hemolysis has occurred with a high-titer anti-B in association with an exchange transfusion of a group B infant.[7-9]

It is important to remember that drug-induced hemolysis may be clinically indistinguishable from AHTR. The hemolysis may be severe and even fatal. Treatment consists of discontinuing the drug, providing supportive care, and administering a transfusion to maintain adequate oxygen-carrying capacity. The cephalosporin antibiotics, cefotetan and ceftriaxone, are now the most common causes of drug-induced immune hemolysis.[10]

Sickle Cell Hemolytic Transfusion Reaction Syndrome

See Alloimmune Cytopenias.

T-Activation of Red Blood Cells

T antigen is a cryptantigen present on glycophorins A and B of the red cell membrane and is not normally exposed on the surface of the red cell. Proteolytic enzymes, produced by certain microorganisms, in particular *Clostridia* species, *Streptococcus pneumoniae*, and influenza viruses, remove sialic acid residues, thereby exposing the T antigen and causing T-activation. T-activation has been reported in infants with sepsis and necrotizing enterocolitis (NEC) and in children with pneumococcal pneumonia.[11,12] All adult plasma and plasma-containing components contain variable amounts of anti-T, which is considered a "naturally occurring" antibody. There have been reports of variable degrees of intravascular hemolysis ranging from none to fatal associated with the passive infusion of anti-T in neonates with T-activation.[7,12] Evidence suggests that mechanisms other than immune hemolysis, such as red cell membrane damage by microbial agents, their products, or both, may play roles in the increased frequency of hemolysis seen in infants with T-activation.[1,7,12] It is difficult to diagnose T-activation during routine compatibility testing; specific agglutination tests with peanut lectin are used.

Opinions vary about the best approach to screening and management.[13] From 10% to 15% of healthy neonates and up to 30% of infants with NEC may exhibit T-activation. Because only a minority develop clinically significant hemolysis, it has been suggested that screening be done only in selected cases.[13] The infants at greatest risk include those with sepsis or NEC with symptoms of hemolysis, particularly after they have received plasma-containing components. Plasma-containing blood components should be used cautiously in infants with clinically significant hemolysis resulting from T-activation, but strict avoidance may be potentially dangerous.[12] Although it is not routine to test donors to obtain low-titer anti-T plasma, some centers follow a protocol of performing a minor crossmatch immediately before transfusion of plasma-containing components. For red cells, additive solution red cells that contain minimal plasma or washed red cells could be used.[13]

Nonimmune Hemolysis

Physical damage to transfused red cells as a result of excessive infusion pressure, overheating, freezing, incompatible intravenous solution, microbial agents, as well as inherent abnormalities of transfused red cells can result in symptoms that mimic an immune-mediated AHTR. Mechanical hemolysis of transfused blood can occur with artificial heart valves, extracorporeal circulation devices, mechanical pumps, and dialysis equipment, as well as during apheresis procedures.[14] Transfusion of red cells through small-gauge needles (≥24 gauge) under high pressure can result in hemolysis because of the stress imposed on erythrocytes, and rapid transfusion should be avoided.

Normal saline is the only compatible fluid to be infused with RBC units. Administration of hypotonic saline solutions, 5% dextrose in water (D5W), distilled water, or certain medications in the same line as the blood infusion can result in osmotic lysis of transfused red cells. Heating above 42 C caused by a malfunctioning blood warmer, or freezing caused by exposure to ice or a refrigerator malfunction, may hemolyze blood before transfusion. Hemolysis of transfused red cells has been reported as a result of blood being administered through the top port of a temperature-controlled neonatal incubator instead of a side port as well as through tubing that crosses the surface of a radiant warmer.[15,16] Red cells deficient in glucose-6 phosphate dehydrogenase (G6PD) are susceptible to hemolysis when exposed to oxidant stress, and donor blood deficient in G6PD has been reported to cause hemolysis in sick neonates.[17] Red cells from donors with sickle cell trait infused in large volume into hypoxic neonates have been reported to cause nonimmune hemolysis.[18,19] It is recommended that blood negative for sickle cell hemoglobin (Hb S) be used when a neonate undergoes massive transfusion[20] (see Special Products). Although hemoglobinuria may occur in nonimmune hemolysis, it is rarely associated with the symptom complex seen with AHTR. Transfusion of hemolyzed blood can cause hyperkalemia and transient renal impairment, as well as hyperbilirubinemia in the neonate. It is important to evaluate the cause of hemoglobinemia, hemoglobinuria, or both as soon as possible, because delay in the recognition of an immune AHTR could lead to serious clinical complications.

Febrile Nonhemolytic Transfusion Reactions

Fever, a common symptom of a transfusion reaction, may be the first sign of a febrile (fever-chill) reaction, bacterial contamination, or AHTR. Fever may also occur as a result of the patient's underlying disease. A febrile nonhemolytic transfusion reaction (FNHTR) is defined as a temperature increase of greater than 1 C (1.8 F) in association with a transfusion, without any other cause. The diagnosis of a FNHTR is one of exclusion. Chills and rigors typically accompany the reactions. Transfusions associated with these symptoms should be stopped and generally should not be restarted because they may be premonitory symptoms of AIHTR, transfusion-related acute lung injury (TRALI), or bacterial contamination. In adults, the FNHTR is the most common acute adverse complication of both red cell and platelet transfusions, with frequencies greater than 30% reported with the latter.[21] Although a FNHTR is usually not observed in infants, children do experience these reactions. The reported frequency, at least in relation to platelet transfusions, is less than in adults, with a frequency of 12% observed in one study with the use of standard platelets.[1,22]

Febrile reactions may be attributed to antibodies present in the recipient's plasma directed against transfused leukocytes, causing release of endogenous pyrogens.[21] Prevention based on this etiology has involved leukocyte reduction of blood components, which has been relatively successful with RBC components. Leukocytes in cellular blood components may produce pyrogens during storage, resulting in a FNHTR in the transfusion recipient. The use of leukocyte-reduced blood components may not necessarily eliminate all of these reactions.[23] Stored blood components, in particular, platelets, have been shown to contain cytokines such as IL-1β, IL-6, IL-8, and TNF-α, which can cause fever during transfusion, independent of the cellular portion of the component.[22,24] The removal of plasma from stored platelets, as well as prestorage leukocyte reduction, can decrease the incidence of febrile reactions secondary to the release of biologic response mediators.[22,25,26] Another postulated mechanism for FNHTR is that during storage platelets release CD40 ligand (CD154), which can stimulate endothelial cells to produce prostaglandin E2 in a manner similar to pyrogenic cytokines.[27]

Most febrile reactions respond to antipyretics (see Table 29). Patients who are thrombocytopenic, however, should not be given aspirin, which interferes with platelet function. While febrile reactions are rarely serious, rigors can be a significant stress for a patient with compromised cardiorespiratory status.

Allergic Reactions

Allergic reactions resulting from the infusion of plasma proteins may cause localized cutaneous manifestations such as urticaria, flushing, and itching to systemic symptoms of nausea, vomiting, diarrhea, and bronchospasm. Allergic reactions are rare in neonates but have been reported to occur in children at a frequency of 5% to 6% with platelet transfusions.[22] These reactions occur when the patient has preformed IgE antibody against an allergen in the donor plasma. Most allergic reactions are mild and do not recur; frank anaphylactic reactions are rare. With mild, localized reactions, the transfusion may be continued after medication has been given, if the symptoms subside. Most reactions respond to oral or parenteral antihistamines.[3]

Anaphylactic reactions can have a very rapid onset, after as little as 10 to 15 mL of a blood component. The severity of the reaction is usually linked to the time interval between the initiation of transfusion and onset of symptoms. Unlike other severe immediate transfusion reactions such as AHTR secondary to ABO incompatibility or septic shock, there is an absence of fever. These reactions are usually caused by antibodies in the recipient, either a potent IgG or IgM, directed against IgA, although antibodies to other proteins such as haptoglobin and C4 (Chido/Rogers blood group antigens) have been implicated.[28-30] For severe allergic or anaphylactic reactions, the transfusion should be stopped immediately, and IV access should be maintained while fluid resuscitation and treatment with epinephrine, steroids, or both are started. Severe reactions may require treatment with vasopressors and intubation. When further red cell transfusions are indicated, the use of washed red cells should be considered. Transfusion of plasma-containing components presents a more difficult problem that requires careful risk/benefit evaluation. Pretransfusion treatment with high-dose corticosteroids and antihistamines should be considered, and epinephrine should be readily available during the transfusion. For IgA-deficient patients with a history of previous severe allergic reaction, anti-IgA, or both, IgA-deficient plasma can be obtained through rare donor registries, if time permits.[3] For any anticipated demand for transfusion, such as future surgery, autologous donations should be considered (see Blood Components).

Circulatory Overload

Large volumes of blood are occasionally transfused to neonates and children in association with acute blood loss, exchange transfusion, extracorporeal membrane oxygenation, and cardiopulmonary bypass surgery. Hypervolemia (circulatory overload) develops when the patient is unable to compensate for expanded blood volume. Infants and children who have preexisting cardiac disease are more susceptible than other pediatric patients. Before transfusion, the estimated volume necessary to achieve the desired hematocrit should be determined (see Adverse Effects of Blood Transfusion) to avoid hypervolemia and polycythemia. Acute hypervolemia resulting from infusion of large volumes of blood in neonates has been associated with cardiopulmonary morbidity and increased risk of intraventricular hemorrhage.[1] Symptoms of circulatory overload in older children may include headache, shortness of breath, pulmonary edema, congestive heart failure, and systolic hypertension. Symptoms usually subside if the transfusion is stopped. It is important to carefully monitor input and output during procedures requiring massive transfusion and to slow infusion rates if clinically warranted. Slower rates of transfusion and diuretics may be needed for children at risk of fluid overload, such as patients with chronic anemia who have an expanded plasma volume or patients with compromised cardiac function, pulmonary function, or both. In these situations, aliquots from a single unit of blood can be transfused slowly over time, not to exceed 4 hours.[3] In addition, some centers will volume-reduce red cell aliquots for transfusion by centrifugation and removal of supernatant. Volume reduction of platelets is not required and may damage platelet function (see Blood Components).

Transfusion-Related Acute Lung Injury

TRALI, a rare but potentially serious adverse effect of transfusion, may be underrecognized. TRALI has occurred in both adults and children as a clinical syndrome manifesting with dyspnea, hypoxia, hypotension, and bilateral pulmonary edema leading to marked opacification of the chest x-ray and fever during or within 4 hours of a transfusion. It is differentiated from circulatory overload because of the absence of heart failure, as well as the lack of response to diuretics. Symptoms usually resolve within 48 to 72 hours; however, in 5% to 10% of cases, TRALI is fatal.

TRALI is the third leading cause of transfusion-related mortality reported to the FDA.[31] It has been associated with the presence of antibodies directed against neutrophil-specific, HLA Class I or Class II antigens and biologically active lipids in the donor plasma.[31,32] The passive transfer of antibodies directed against recipient leukocytes has been associated with a spectrum of acute lung injuries that manifest as acute pulmonary edema. This reaction results from activation of recipient neutrophils in the lungs with the production of vasoactive mediators, ultimately causing capillary leakage. The donor of the implicated unit is often a multiparous woman.[31] Less commonly, recipient antibodies directed against donor leukocytes are implicated as a cause of TRALI. The transfusion of leukocyte-reduced components may be beneficial in this setting. A test for HLA and neutrophil-specific antibodies in both donor and recipient may help establish the diagnosis.[3]

Alternatively, a lipid mediator produced by donor leukocytes during storage may prime recipient neutrophils so that a second stimulus, such as inflammation, infection, or tissue injury, results in the release of vasoactive mediators (the two-hit hypothesis).[33]

The treatment of TRALI is supportive and consists of maintenance of ventilation and hemodynamic status. The patient may require supplemental oxygen, endotracheal intubation, and respiratory support until the intra-alveolar fluid can be resorbed. Diuresis is not indicated. Steroids may shorten the course of TRALI, but their role in therapy is unclear. Fluid support may be necessary for resuscitation in the event of hypotension and marked movement of fluid from plasma to the extravascular space.

Bacterial Contamination

Bacterial contamination of stored blood and blood components poses a rare but serious risk to the transfusion recipient and is the most common cause of death from infectious disease reported to the FDA from 1990 to 1998. Although both red cell and platelet components have been implicated, contaminated platelet concentrates have been responsible for a larger proportion of fatal cases.[34] Bacteria can enter a blood bag because of improper preparation of the skin at the venipuncture site at the time of phlebotomy, because of improper component preparation or handling, or because of occult bacteremia in the donor. Skin flora (*Staphylococci, Propionibacteria*) are the most common isolates from prospectively cultured units, but gram-negative rods (*Acinetobacter, Klebsiella, Escherichia*) and gram-positive cocci (*Staphylococcus, Streptococcus*) have been implicated in clinical reactions to contaminated red cells and platelets.[34,35] Bacteria capable of growing at low temperature in a high-iron environment, such as *Yersinia* or *Pseudo-*

monas, may proliferate in RBC units that are stored in refrigerators.

The clinical symptoms associated with bacterially contaminated components depend on the type of organism present. In the case of gram-negative organisms that produce endotoxin, the patient may develop rigors, high fever, dyspnea, hypotension, and shock. Hemoglobinemia and hemoglobinuria are usually absent. The transfusion must be stopped immediately when a contaminated unit is suspected, and treatment should include a culture, intravenous antibiotics, and appropriate care for endotoxic shock.

Suspected septic transfusion reactions should be reported to the transfusion service because additional components collected from the same donation could be infected and must be recalled. On occasion, septic reactions may not manifest until several hours after the transfusion of a unit of contaminated blood.[3] To document a septic reaction, cultures from the blood component and the patient's blood must grow the same organism. Because patients may already be on antibiotics, their cultures may be negative. Efforts to screen platelet components for bacteria are under way.[35] Whole blood collection bags with a diversion pouch have been shown to reduce contamination with skin flora.[36]

Thermal Effects

Infants and children are predisposed to hypothermia because of their large surface-area-to-weight ratio. Hypothermia can result in decreased oxygen delivery to tissues secondary to a leftward shift in the oxyhemoglobin dissociation curve.[37] In adults, the rapid transfusion of blood directly from refrigerator storage has resulted in hypothermia-induced cardiac arrest.[38] The transfusion of cold blood in neonates has been associated with apnea and hypoglycemia.[37] Conversely, over-warming blood can produce hemolysis; blood should be warmed using only a monitored blood-warming system.

Metabolic Complications

The immature development of several organ systems in premature infants places them at increased risk of metabolic complications that could be potentiated by the administration of blood, particularly in association with massive transfusion or exchange transfusion. Blood is anticoagulated with citrate, which chelates calcium ions. Rapid or massive transfusion can result in a transient decrease in ionized calcium levels.[39] Fresh Frozen Plasma and Whole Blood are the blood components most likely to cause hypocalcemia because they contain the most citrate per unit volume.[37] Symptomatic hypocalcemia is rare, and calcium supplementation is rarely required. Classic signs of peripheral motor nerve hyperexcitability are uncommon in infants. Clinical manifestations in the neonate undergoing exchange transfusion are subtle and variable and include jitteriness, apnea, cyanosis, poor feeding, lethargy, and seizures.[7] There also may be a prolongation of the QT interval, and careful cardiac monitoring will aid in avoiding citrate toxicity during large-volume transfusion. Under no circumstances should calcium be added to a unit of blood because it could reverse the anticoagulant effect of the citrate, producing large blood clots.

The reversible leakage of potassium into the supernatant that occurs during storage of RBCs is enhanced when RBC units are irradiated. The risk of developing hyperkalemia depends on the patient's size and clinical condition, the type and amount of component transfused, the concentration of plasma potassium (age dependent), and the rate and route of infusion. Although the potassium concentration may be high in stored units of blood, the total amount infused in a small-volume transfusion usually is not clinically significant.

As an example, a small-volume transfusion of 15 mL/kg of an additive solution RBC unit with a hematocrit of 56% and plasma potassium of 50 mEq/L (amount at outdate of unit—42 days) to a 1-kg infant over 3 hours would result in the infusion of 0.11 mEq of potassium/kg/hour. This rate would come close to the infant's daily requirement of 2 to 3 mEq/kg/day. However, hyperkalemia caused by the massive infusion of stored blood may occur. In this setting, infusion occurs much more rapidly, and the infusion may be into a central line instead of a peripheral line. Hyperkalemia reduces transmembrane potential, resulting in delayed depolarization, faster repolarization, and reduction of conduction velocity. Infants may show signs of muscular weakness and ileus. Cardiac arrhythmias are not uncommon, and fatal arrhythmias have been associated with massive transfusion.[40]

Washing of RBC units, removal of the supernatant, or use of fresh blood (ie, less than 7 to 14 days old) should be considered in clinical situations in which the patients are at risk of developing hyperkalemia. These scenarios include the presence of pre-existing hyperkalemia or renal failure, the need for rapid or bolus administration of blood, the administration of large-volume transfusions (>20 mL/kg or exchange transfusion), or the use of direct cardiac administration.

Both hypoglycemia and hyperglycemia have been reported in association with transfusion in the neonate.[7] Glucose production in the neonate correlates directly with brain and body mass. Glucose turnover, when related to body mass, greatly exceeds that of adults. Hypoglycemia during transfusion may occur as a result of a decreased infusion of glucose if all sources of intravenous fluid are discontinued during transfusion. Hypoglycemia is usually asymptomatic and may go unrecognized during routine transfusion if the infant is not monitored. Hypoglycemic episodes are more frequently observed with transfusions of CPDA-1 RBCs than additive solution RBCs.[41] Hypoglycemia that occurs in association with exchange transfusion is the result of a high glucose load that stimulates endogenous insulin and results in a rebound hypoglycemia. Premature infants may also be less tolerant of the increased glucose loads of large-volume transfusion, particularly when anesthesia is required for surgical procedures. Anesthesia may induce the release of epinephrine and mobilization of endogenous glucose stores.[7]

Delayed Transfusion Reactions

Alloimmunization

See Alloimmune Cytopenias.

Delayed Hemolytic Reactions

Delayed hemolytic transfusion reactions (DHTRs) occur when antigens carried on transfused red cells induce an antibody response in a recipient, usually 4 to 7 days (anamnestic response) or several weeks (primary response) after the transfusion episode. Most antibodies associated with DHTRs are IgG, rarely fix complement, and result in extravascular hemolysis in the spleen and, to a lesser extent, in the liver. The coating of the transfused donor red cells with recipient antibodies will cause a positive DAT result. Usually, DHTRs manifest as slight fever, malaise, weakness, and symptoms referable to anemia. Other laboratory findings may include an elevated reticulocyte count, increased indirect bilirubin and lactate dehydrogenase, or normal or slightly decreased haptoglobin. Spherocytes may be observed on blood smears. Hemoglobinemia is unusual.

Delayed intravascular hemolytic transfusion reactions may occur and are most often associated with antibodies to the Duffy or Kidd blood group antigen systems. Although complement is activated to C5-9 component and hemolysis with hemoglobinemia and hemoglobinuria may occur, the rate of generation of biologic response modifiers is lower than in an AIHTR.[5] Most of these reactions are not life threatening; however, severe hemolysis, although rare, can occur. If a patient shows signs of a severe transfusion reaction, treatment should follow that described for an AIHTR.

Posttransfusion Purpura

See Alloimmune Cytopenias.

Transfusion-Associated Graft-vs-Host Disease

Transfusion-associated graft-vs-host disease (TA-GVHD) occurs when immunocompetent T lymphocytes are infused into a recipient, are not rejected, recognize host histocompatibility antigens as foreign, and attack host tissue. This complication of transfusion, usually associated with an immunoincompetent recipient, has also been observed after transfusion of cellular components from HLA-homozygous donors to immunocompetent recipients who are heterozygous for the HLA haplotype.[42] Although the latter occurs more frequently after transfusion of blood from first- or second-degree relatives, it has been reported to occur with transfusion of blood from unrelated HLA-homozygous donors.[43]

TA-GVHD typically begins 8 to 10 days after transfusion and is characterized by fever, followed 24 to 48 hours later by a central maculopapular skin rash that spreads to the extremities. Diarrhea, hepatitis, and marrow aplasia are also part of the symptom complex. Dysregulation of cytokines is the primary cause of induction and maintenance of TA-GVHD.[44] TA-GVHD is fatal in most cases, usually as a result of overwhelming infection or bleeding secondary to marrow failure. The median time to death is approximately 21 days. In neonates, the onset to symptoms is longer, approximately 28 days, with a median time to death of 51 days.[45]

Because the symptoms associated with TA-GVHD can be observed with viral syndromes, sepsis, and drug reactions or be obscured by comorbid conditions, one has to have a high index of suspicion. A definitive diagnosis of TA-GVHD relies on showing the persistence of donor lymphocytes in the recipient's peripheral circulation or affected tissues. TA-GVHD can be prevented by gamma irradiation of cellular blood components, which renders donor lymphocytes incapable of proliferating.[46] To prevent TA-GVHD in susceptible patients (see Special Products), blood and cellular components must be irradiated with at least 2500 cGy.[20]

Hemosiderosis

One mL of red cells contains 1 mg of iron. Because there is no physiologic mechanism for the excretion of excess iron, children with chronic anemia (ie, thalassemia) requiring long-term transfusion therapy will develop iron overload over time. Accumulation of iron eventually produces organ damage, particularly in the heart, liver, and pancreas. The parenteral iron chelator desferoxamine can prevent the complications of iron overload in patients receiving chronic red cell transfusion therapy.[47] Red cell exchange by apheresis has been used to limit iron accumulation in patients with sickle cell disease who require repeated transfusions (see Alloimmune Cytopenias).

Plasticizer and Lead Exposure

Polyvinyl chloride (PVC) compounds are used in a wide array of medical devices, including blood bags and intravenous tubing. These plastics are made flexible through the addition of plasticizers, the most common being di-2-ethylhexyl phthalate (DEHP). DEHP is a lyphophilic compound, which has been shown to leach into biologic fluids containing lipid, such as all blood components. The concentration present in a blood bag depends on the temperature, duration of storage, and composition of the component.[48] DEHP is metabolized to mono-(2-ethylhexyl)-phthalate and is rapidly excreted by the kidneys in healthy individuals. Certain populations of patients, such as those on dialysis, may have chronic exposure to these compounds; other populations, such as neonates and fetuses, may have exposure during critical times of development. Toxicologic studies in animals and in-vitro studies have linked exposure to DEHP and metabolites to adverse effects on the infant liver, kidneys, heart, lungs, and reproductive system, as well as fetal effects.[1,48,49] The developing testis may be more susceptible to the testicular toxicity of DEHP. Although high levels of DEHP have been observed in infants undergoing exchange transfusion and extracorporeal membrane oxygenation, no evidence of toxicity has been reported to date.[49] However, epidemiologic studies of DEHP exposure in humans are not available, and further research is warranted before changes in transfusion recommendations can be made.

An association has been established between the exposure of low-to-moderate levels of lead in early childhood and modest declines in psychometric intelligence.[50] Recent data have shown that blood transfusions represent a source of lead exposure for premature infants.[51] Further investigation is necessary before definitive recommendations for routine screening of banked blood for lead levels could be entertained.

Transfusion-Transmitted Diseases

Despite extensive donor screening and increased testing, infections still may be transmitted by blood transfusion. Most transmissions of hepatitis or human immunodeficiency virus (HIV) occur from donors in the "window period" between infection and appearance of detectable antibody or virus.[52] (See Table 30.) All cases of suspected posttransfusion infection should be reported to the blood bank to facilitate the identification of infectious donors and to prevent further transmissions.

Hepatitis

Hepatitis C virus (HCV) accounts for the majority of post-transfusion hepatitis, most of which was acquired before the im-

Table 30. Current Estimated Viral Window-Period Risk in American Red Cross Repeat Blood Donor Population[52]

Virus	Screening Markers	Window Period (Days)	Risk (Rate Infectious Donations)
HIV-1/2	Anti-HIV and p24	16	1:1,468,000
HIV-1/2	Anti-HIV and NAT	11	1:2,135,000
HTLV-I/II	Anti-HTLV	51	1:2,993,000
HCV	Anti-HCV and NAT	10	1:1,935,000
HBV	HBsAg	59	1:205,000

HIV = human immunodeficiency virus; HTLV = human T-cell lymphotropic virus; HCV = hepatitis C virus; NAT = nucleic acid amplification testing; HBV = hepatitis B virus; HBsAg = hepatitis B surface antigen.

plementation of serologic screening. In adults, acquired infection persists in up to 70% to 80% of patients, who are usually asymptomatic. Cirrhosis develops within 20 years in approximately 20% of infected individuals; approximately 10% of patients with cirrhosis develop hepatocellular carcinoma. In children, the course of transfusion-associated HCV may vary depending on the underlying disease. It has been suggested that transfusion-acquired HCV early in childhood may resolve without treatment more commonly than infection acquired later in life.[53,54]

In contrast to HCV, acute hepatitis B virus (HBV) infection is symptomatic in 30% to 50% of adults but in less than 10% of children who are less than 5 years old. Chronic infection occurs in 2% to 10% of adults but in 30% to 90% of children who are less than 5 years old. Premature death from cirrhosis or hepatocellular carcinoma occurs in 15% to 25% of chronic carriers.[3] Estimates of the per-unit risk of transfusion-transmitted hepatitis are 1:205,000 for HBV and 1:1,935,000 for HCV in repeat donors.[52] The rates in first-time donors are twice as high. The risk of HCV transmission has declined dramatically since the introduction of nucleic acid amplification testing (NAT) in 1999. Hepatitis A transmission has occurred with plasma derivatives, but it is not a substantial risk for blood components.

HIV

Transfusion-transmitted HIV has declined markedly since the implementation of antibody testing in 1985. The clinical manifestations of transfusion-transmitted HIV infection are similar to those of infections acquired through other routes. The rapidity with which the recipient progresses to AIDS is independent of donor status. Although the current transmission rate by transfusion is very low, new cases continue to be discovered resulting from past transfusions, usually through the look-back process of identifying recipients of blood from a donor subsequently diagnosed with HIV. Current donor screening tests include NAT for HIV. The per-unit risk of HIV transmission is estimated to be 1:2,135,000, although it is difficult to be precise with such a low incidence.[52]

Cytomegalovirus

See Special Products.

Other Viruses

Human T-cell lymphotrophic viruses (HTLV-I/II) are retroviruses unrelated to HIV and are rare in the United States. They are associated with adult T-cell lymphoma/leukemia and peripheral neuropathy (HTLV-associated myelopathy, HAM). Parvovirus B19 causes erythema infectiosum in childhood. This virus can infect red cell precursors in the marrow and, in patients with accelerated hematopoiesis (eg, sickle cell disease), can cause hypoplastic or aplastic anemia. Although parvovirus B19 is common in the general population and transmission by blood transfusion occurs, it seldom causes significant disease.[55] Epstein-Barr virus, which is transmissible by transfusion, appears to be of clinical significance only in immunocompromised transfusion recipients. Transfusion-transmitted West Nile virus (WNV) has occurred in the United States, with a risk of approximately 1 to 3/10,000 units.[56] Transmission has occurred in association with RBCs, platelets, and Fresh Frozen Plasma. NAT screening for WNV began in July 2003.

Parasites

Transfusion-transmitted malaria occurs in the United States but is uncommon.[57] The mortality rate of transfusion-transmitted malaria is 10%, with the most frequent species implicated being *Plasmodium falciparum*. Exclusion of donors on the basis of geographic risk factors is the most effective preventive measure. *Babesia microti* is widely distributed in North America where transfusion-transmitted babesiosis has been reported.[58] It presently is the most common transfusion-transmitted parasitic infection in the United States and has been transmitted by transfusion in infants.[59] Current serologic tests are inadequate for blood donor screening. Transfusion transmission of *Trypanosoma cruzi*, the cause of Chagas' disease, is a significant problem in areas of the world where the causative agent is endemic, but it has occurred rarely in the United States. Serologic screening for *T. cruzi* infection may be effective where a high proportion of donors have emigrated from such areas, but it is not performed on blood collected in the United States.[3]

Prions

Creutzfeldt-Jakob disease (CJD) is a degenerative brain disorder caused by an infection with proteinaceous particles known as prions. Variant CJD (vCJD) differs from classic CJD in lack of affected family members, younger age of onset, more rapid progression, and association with consumption of certain animal products. No cases of CJD or vCJD transmission by blood transfusion have been reported; however, experimental models suggest that transmission by blood components is possible.[60] B cells and dendritic cells may play a crucial role in the development of spongiform encephalopathy, which has led to the adoption of leukocyte reduction to minimize the risk of transfusion-transmitted vCJD.[61] However, no data exist demonstrating that universal leukocyte reduction is efficacious in preventing the spread of vCJD by transfused blood. Because no practical donor screening test for the abnormal isoform of the prion protein is available, the current strategies for reducing the theoretical risk of transmission include deferring donors with a family history of CJD, exposure to certain known risk factors, or residence or extended travel in regions where vCJD is endemic.[3]

References

1. Holman P, Blajchman MA, Heddle N. Noninfectious adverse effects of blood transfusion in the neonate. Transfus Med Rev 1995;9:277-87.
2. Siberry GK, Iannone R, eds. The Harriet Lane handbook. 15th ed. St Louis, MO: Mosby Publishing Co., 2000.

3. Triulzi DJ, ed. Blood transfusion therapy: A physician's handbook. 7th ed. Bethesda, MD: American Association of Blood Banks, 2002.
4. Sazama K. Reports of 355 transfusion associated deaths 1976 through 1985. Transfusion 1990;30:583-90.
5. Davenport RD. Hemolytic transfusion reactions. In: Popovsky MA, ed. Transfusion reactions. 2nd ed. Bethesda, MD: AABB Press, 2001:1-64.
6. Pawloski JR, Stamler JS. Nitric oxide in RBCs. Transfusion 2002;42:1603-9.
7. Pisciotto PT, Luban NLC. Complications of neonatal transfusion. In: Popovsky MA, ed. Transfusion reactions. 2nd ed. Bethesda, MD: AABB Press, 2001:359-94.
8. Pierce RN, Reich LM, Mayer K. Hemolysis following platelet transfusions from ABO-incompatible donors. Transfusion 1985;25:60-2.
9. Kim HC, Park CL, Cowan JH, et al. Massive intravascular hemolysis associated with intravenous immunoglobulin in bone marrow transplant recipients. Am J Pediatr Hematol Oncol 1988;10:69-74.
10. Arndt PA, Leger RM, Garratty G. Serology of antibodies to second- and third-generation cephalosporins associated with immune hemolytic anemia and/or positive direct antiglobulin tests. Transfusion 1999;39:1239-46.
11. Williams RA, Brown EF, Hurst D, Franklin LC. Transfusion of infants with activation of erythrocyte T antigen. J Pediatr 1989;115:949-53.
12. Eder AF, Manno CS. Does red-cell T activation matter? Annotation. Br J Haematol 2001;114:25-30.
13. Engelfriet CP, Reesink HW. Blood transfusion in premature or young infants with polyagglutination and activation of the T antigen. Vox Sang 1999;76:128-32.
14. Beauregard P, Blajchman MA. Hemolytic and pseudohemolytic transfusion reactions: An overview of the hemolytic transfusion reactions and the clinical conditions that mimic them. Transfus Med Rev 1994;8:184-99.
15. Opitz JC, Baldauf MC, Kessler DL, et al. Hemolysis of blood in intravenous tubing caused by heat. J Pediatr 1987;112:111-13.

16. Strauss RG, Bell EF, Snyder EL, et al. Effects of environmental warming on blood components dispensed in syringes for neonatal transfusions. J Pediatr 1986;109:109-13.
17. Mimouni F, Shohat S, Reisner SH. G6PD deficient donor blood as a cause of haemolysis in two preterm infants. Isr J Med Sci 1986;22:120-2.
18. Murphy RJC, Malhotra C, Swet AY. Death following an exchange transfusion with hemoglobin SC blood. J Pediatr 1980;96:110-12.
19. Veiga S, Vaithianathan T. Massive intravascular sickling after exchange transfusion with sickle cell trait blood. Transfusion 1963;3:387-91.
20. Fridey JL, ed. Standards for blood banks and transfusion services. 22nd ed. Bethesda, MD: American Association of Blood Banks, 2003:51.
21. Heddle NM, Kelton JG. Febrile nonhemolytic transfusion reactions. In: Popovsky MA, ed. Transfusion reactions. 2nd ed. Bethesda, MD: AABB Press, 2001:45-82.
22. Couban S, Carruthers J, Andreou P, et al. Platelet transfusions in children: Results of a randomized, prospective, crossover trial of plasma removal and a prospective audit of WBC reduction. Transfusion 2002;42:753-8.
23. Mangano MM, Chambers LA, Kruskall MS. Limited efficacy of leukopoor platelets for prevention of febrile transfusion reactions. Am J Clin Pathol 1991;95:733-8.
24. Heddle NM, Klama L, Singer J, et al. The role of the plasma from platelet concentrates in transfusion reactions. N Engl J Med 1994;331:625-8.
25. Heddle NM, Blajchman MA, Meyer RM, et al. A randomized controlled trial comparing the frequency of acute reactions to plasma-removed platelets and prestorage WBC-reduced platelets. Transfusion 2002;42:556-66.
26. Uhlmann EJ, Isgriggs E, Wallhermfechtel M, Goodnough LT. Prestorage universal WBC reduction of RBC units does not affect the incidence of transfusion reactions. Transfusion 2001;41:997-1000.
27. Phipps RP, Kaufman J, Blumberg N. Platelet derived CD154 (CD40 ligand) and febrile responses to transfusion. Lancet 2001;357:2023-4.

28. Sandler SG, Mallory D, Malamut D, Eckrich R. IgA anaphylactic transfusion reactions. Transfus Med Rev 1995;9:1-8.
29. Westhoff CM, Sipherd BD, Wylie DE, Toalson LD. Severe anaphylactic reaction following transfusion of platelets to a patient with anti-Ch. Transfusion 1992;32:576-9.
30. Koda Y, Watanabe Y, Soejima M, et al. Simple PCR detection of haptoglobin gene deletion in anhaptoglobinemic patients with antihaptoglobin antibody that causes anaphylactic transfusion reactions. Blood 2000;95:1138-43.
31. Popovsky MA. Transfusion-related acute lung injury. In: Popovsky MA, ed. Transfusion reactions. 2nd ed. Bethesda, MD: AABB Press, 2001:155-70.
32. Kopko PM, Marshall CS, MacKenzie MR, et al. Transfusion-related acute lung injury: Report of a clinical look-back investigation. JAMA 2002;287:1968-71.
33. Silliman CC, Paterson AJ, Dickey WO, et al. The association of biologically active lipids with the development of transfusion-related acute lung injury: A retrospective study. Transfusion 1997;37:719-26.
34. Kuehnart MJ, Roth VR, Haley NR, et al. Transfusion-transmitted bacterial infection in the United States: 1998-2000. Transfusion 2001;41:1493-9.
35. Dodd RY, Lipton KS. Guidance on implementation of new bacteria reduction and detection standard. Association Bulletin #03-07. Bethesda, MD: American Association of Blood Banks, 2003.
36. Bruneau C, Perez P, Chassaigne M, et al. Efficacy of a new collection procedure for preventing bacterial contamination of whole-blood donations. Transfusion 2001;41:74-81.
37. Barcelona SL, Cote CJ. Pediatric resuscitation in the operating room. Anesthesiol Clin North Am 2001;19:339-65.
38. Boyan CP, Howland WS. Cardiac arrest and temperature of blood bank blood. N Engl J Med 1963;183:58-60.
39. Jackson JC. Adverse events associated with exchange transfusion in healthy and ill newborns. Pediatrics 1997;99:E7.

40. Hall TL, Barnes A, Miller JR, et al. Neonatal mortality following transfusion of red cells with high plasma potassium levels. Transfusion 1993;33:606-9.
41. Goodstein MH, Locke RG, Wlodarczyk D, et al. Comparison of two preservation solutions for erythrocyte transfusions in newborn infants. J Pediatr 1993;123:783-8.
42. Linden JV, Pisciotto PT. Transfusion-associated graft-versus-host disease and blood irradiation. Transfus Med Rev 1992;6:116-23.
43. Shivdasani RA, Haluska FG, Dock NL, et al. Graft-versus-host disease associated with transfusion of blood from unrelated HLA-homozygous donors. N Engl J Med 1993; 328:766-70.
44. Ferrara JM, Kreger W. Graft-versus-host disease: The influence of type 1 and type 2 T cell cytokines. Transfus Med Rev 1998;33:742-50.
45. Ohto H, Anderson KC. Posttransfusion graft-versus-host disease in immunocompetent recipients. Transfusion 1996;36:117-23.
46. Moroff G, Luban NLC. The irradiation of blood and blood components to prevent graft-versus-host disease: Technical issues and guidelines. Transfus Med Rev 1997;11:15-26.
47. Giardina PJ, Grady RW. Chelation therapy in β-thalassemia: An optimistic update. Semin Hematol 2001;38: 360-6.
48. Tickner JA, Schettler T, Guidotti T, et al. Health risks posed by use of di-2-ethylhexyl phthalate (DEHP) in PVC medical devices: A critical review. Am J Ind Med 2001; 39:100-11.
49. Latini G. Potential hazards of exposure to di-(2- ethylhexyl)-phthalate in babies. Biol Neonate 2000;78: 269-76.
50. Cranfield RL, Henderson CR, Cory-Slechta DA, et al. Intellectual impairment in children with blood lead concentrations below 10 mg per deciliter. N Engl J Med 2003; 348:1517-26.
51. Bearer CF, O'Riordan MA, Powers R. Lead exposure from blood transfusion to premature infants. J Pediatr 2000;137:549-54.

52. Dodd R, Notari EP, Stramer SL. Current prevalence and incidence of infectious disease markers and estimated window-period risk in the American Red Cross blood donor population. Transfusion 2002;42:975-9.
53. Minola E, Prati D, Suter F, et al. Age at infection affects the long-term outcome of transfusion-associated chronic hepatitis C. Blood 2002;99:4588-91.
54. Vogt M, Lang T, Frosner G, et al. Prevalence and clinical outcome of hepatitis C infection in children who underwent cardiac surgery before the implementation of blood-donor screening. N Engl J Med 1999;341:866-70.
55. Koenigbauer UF, Eastland T, Day JW. Clinical illness due to parvovirus B19 infection after infusion of solvent/detergent-treated pooled plasma. Transfusion 2000;40:1203-6.
56. Biggerstaff BJ, Petersen LR. Estimated risk of West Nile virus transmission through blood transfusion during an epidemic in Queens, New York City. Transfusion 2002;42:1019-26.
57. Mungai M, Tegtmeier G, Chamberland M, Parise M. Transfusion-transmitted malaria in the United States from 1963 through 1999. N Engl J Med 2001;344:1973-8.
58. Leiby DA, Chung APS, Cable RG, et al. Relationship between tick bites and the seroprevalence of *Babesia microti* and *Anaplasma phagocytophilia* (previously *Ehrlichia* sp.) in blood donors. Transfusion 2002;42:1585-91.
59. Dobroszycki J, Herwaldt BL, Boctor F, et al. A cluster of transfusion-associated babesiosis cases traced to a single asymptomatic donor. JAMA 1999;281:927-30.
60. Houston F, Foster JD, Chong A, et al. Transmission of BSE by blood transfusion in sheep. Lancet 2000;356:999-1000.
61. Klein MA, Frigg R, Flechsig E, et al. A crucial role for B cells in neuroinvasive scrapie. Nature 1997;390:687-9.

SPECIAL PRODUCTS

Overview of Special Products

The intent of many regulations pertaining to donor questioning and testing; to blood and blood component collection policies; and to the storage, issuance, and infusion of blood components is to ensure transfusion safety. Despite these general measures, additional complications of blood transfusion pose potential risks to infants and to children with underlying hematologic, oncologic, and immunologic disorders. Examples include cytomegalovirus (CMV) infection, graft-vs-host-disease (GVHD), immunologic responses to transfused leukocytes, and, in the setting of massive red cell replacement, significant accumulation of red cells containing sickle hemoglobin when blood is collected from donors with sickle cell trait. As discussed in the following sections, the term "special products" refers to blood components collected, processed, or selected specifically to minimize these complications.

CMV-Reduced-Risk Components

CMV is a ubiquitous virus with most people becoming infected as children or young adults—generally, via exposure to respiratory secretions. Primary infection with CMV begins as an acute upper respiratory infection, often subclinical, and, as with other herpes viruses, is followed by a "latent" state of chronic infection during which the patient appears well—unless reactivation infection occurs. In healthy individuals, CMV infection is of little consequence, but in patients with immunodeficiency (Table 31), it can be severe, even fatal. During the latent stage of CMV infection, normal individuals are healthy and can donate blood. In the bloodstream of individuals with latent infection, CMV seems to be associated with leukocytes, but the subpopulation carrying the virus has been debated.

Patients at Risk

It is reasonable to predict that removal of the vast majority of leukocytes from cellular blood components collected from seropositive donors (ie, those with serum antibody to CMV) or from untested donors (ie, CMV antibody status unknown) would decrease transmission of CMV to seronegative recipients. All seronegative (ie, no serum antibody to CMV) pediatric patients at risk of severe CMV infection (Table 31) should receive blood components known to pose minimal risk for transfusion-transmitted CMV. Although rare seropositive patients have acquired second primary infections with new strains of CMV, transfusion-transmitted CMV secondary infections have not been reported in seropositive patients. Thus, transfusion of blood components with minimal risk of transmitting CMV is not recommended for seropositive patients[1]—with the important exception of infants during the first 4 to 6 months of life. During this time, it is common practice to give both seronegative and seropositive infants blood components with

Table 31. Patients at Risk for Severe CMV Infection

- Congenital immunodeficiency disorders
- AIDS (human immunodeficiency virus infection)
- Hematopoietic progenitor cell transplant recipients
- Organ allograft transplant recipients
- Premature infants during infancy
- Cancer patients undergoing intense chemotherapy
- Recipients of intrauterine transfusions

minimal risk of CMV. This is because seropositive infants will lose CMV antibodies during the first months of life because they nearly always acquire maternal antibodies via the placenta and have not been truly infected with CMV.

Thus, maternal antibody will be catabolized over time and will decrease to levels in the infant's plasma that do not afford protection from transfusion-transmitted CMV. Also, infants who are seropositive due to maternal antibody, in the absence of true infection, will have no cell-mediated immunity against CMV. Thus, all newborn infants may be at risk for transfusion-transmitted CMV—whether or not they test positive for CMV antibody. Although the clinical manifestations of CMV infection in preterm infants can be severe, there are few convincing data that seronegative full-term infants require blood components with low risk of CMV or that giving CMV-reduced-risk components to seropositive infants of any gestational age truly offers benefit.

Clinical Significance

The clinical importance of transfusion-transmitted CMV in neonates is controversial. Some studies conducted during the 1970s and 1980s reported a disturbingly high incidence (25% to 50%) of CMV, often with organ dysfunction, in infants transfused with cellular blood components,[2] whereas, others suggested a negligible risk.[3] Regardless of the controversy, once a physician or an institution decides to transfuse blood components with a minimal risk of transmitting CMV, cellular blood components should either be obtained from donors who are seronegative for antibody to CMV or effectively leukocyte-reduced.[4] Cellular blood components that have been leukocyte-reduced to a level of $<5 \times 10^6$ WBCs per unit offer safety comparable to that of blood products supplied by seronegative donors.[1,4] Frozen deglycerolized Red Blood Cells (RBCs) are used by some centers and pose little, if any, risk of CMV.[5] However, frozen RBCs are not recommended for general transfusion support for neonates because they offer no clear benefits. Additionally, they are expensive and red cell loss is unavoidable during deglycerolization (ie, up to 20% of red cells are lost)—a situation that could lead to increased donor exposure.

Frozen plasma products (Fresh Frozen Plasma and Cryoprecipitated AHF) are not known to transmit CMV; they do not have to be obtained from seronegative donors nor leukocyte-reduced.[6]

Prevention

Prevention of CMV by leukocyte reduction has been extensively studied,[7] and it is clear that the risk of infection with this virus can be strikingly reduced by consistently removing leukocytes from cellular blood components such as RBC and platelet units. Although all leukocyte reduction studies have been strikingly successful, they are not scientifically "perfect." As noted by Strauss,[7] not all studies were controlled, only a few studies focused on the use of leukocyte reduction to prevent CMV infections specifically during infancy, and the extent of leukocyte reduction was not always clearly stated. The precise dose of WBCs known to transmit CMV is unknown, but transfusions that contain $<5 \times 10^6$ WBCs/unit are extremely unlikely to be infectious.

As an alternative to leukocyte reduction, the rate of transfusion-associated CMV has been reduced by selecting blood components collected from seronegative donors (ie, no serum antibody to CMV). However, this alternative is not perfect. A rate of 1% to 4% CMV infection—as measured by CMV antibody seroconversion, viremia, or viruria—has been reported after transfusion of CMV-seronegative components.[1,7,8] This finding can be attributed to: 1) imperfect sensitivity of tests to detect antibody to CMV; 2) decrease in donor antibody titer over time to levels below limit of detection; 3) transient viremia that quenches circulating antibody; and 4) false-negative result during the early preantibody "window" phase of donor primary infection.

Although some physicians would prefer more convincing data, it is reasonable to conclude that leukocyte reduction of cellular blood components (eg, RBCs and platelets) by any method capable of consistently achieving a residual WBC count of <1 to 5×10^6/unit reduces the risk of transfusion-transmitted CMV to a level similar to that of CMV-seronegative components. Recently, the rate of CMV infection—defined by detection of

CMV antigenemia—was increased in CMV-seronegative progenitor cell transplant recipients, who received large numbers of CMV-reduced-risk blood components including both CMV seronegative and leukocyte-reduced components, when compared to historical control patients.[9] This increase emphasizes that "breakthrough" CMV infections will continue to occur regardless of current methods to reduce risks. Although first collecting blood components from CMV-seronegative donors and then removing the WBCs, theoretically, might improve safety, no data are available to document the efficacy of this combined approach. Until data have established its efficacy, this approach is not recommended because it limits blood availability and is extremely costly without providing known benefit.

Gamma-Irradiated Components

The intent of γ-irradiating cellular blood components is to prevent GVHD mediated by T lymphocytes in units of RBCs, platelets, and granulocytes (ie, neutrophils). Although GVHD has been prevented by other methods such as ultraviolet irradiation, extreme leukocyte reduction, and techniques of pathogen inactivation that damage lymphocyte nucleic acids, these methods are experimental and not approved for standard clinical practice. The indications for γ-irradiated blood components for older infants and children are identical to those for adults (Table 32).

Patients at Risk

Neonates, particularly those who are extremely preterm, are at risk for transfusion-associated GVHD. However, the extent to which they are at risk and the need, or lack thereof, to transfuse γ-irradiated cellular blood components are controversial questions for which no irrefutable, scientifically proven answers exist. Although the immune system of infants unquestionably exhibits diminished function when compared to the immunity of older children and adults, results of immunologic studies in neonates are

Table 32. Patients Who Should Receive Gamma-Irradiated Blood Components*

- Congenital immunodeficiency disorders of cellular immunity
- Intrauterine or neonatal exchange transfusions
- Hematopoietic progenitor cell transplant recipients
- Recipients of blood components from blood-related donors
- HLA-matched cellular blood components
- Hematologic malignancies and Hodgkin's disease
- Cancer patients undergoing intense chemotherapy or receiving fludarabine

*Patients for whom recommendations are controversial include organ allograft recipients, those with AIDS or aplastic anemia with severe lymphocytopenia, premature infants during infancy, and infants undergoing extracorporeal membrane oxygenation.

quite variable. Findings in infant blood include normal or decreased T lymphocytes, normal or increased T4 lymphocytes, normal or decreased T8 lymphocytes leading to an increased T4:T8 ratio, presence of "immature" T lymphocytes, increased B lymphocytes, and decreased natural killer cells. Functional studies reveal normal proliferation of peripheral blood mononuclear cells in response to mitogens, but decreased cytotoxicity and cytokine production. As another confounding factor, the "immunomodulatory" effects of clinical conditions such as infection, nutritional status, surgery, or multiple transfusions further alter immune function. For example, the T4:T8 ratio (ie, CD4:CD8) in infant blood has been reported to be inversely related to the number of transfusions given due to a posttransfusion increase of T8 lymphocytes. Also, a posttransfusion increase in activated T lymphocytes has been reported. Thus, the degree of defective immunologic function of individual neonates requiring transfusions is difficult to predict accurately—as is the risk, or lack thereof, of developing transfusion-associated GVHD.

In an earlier literature review,[7] 73 infants were identified with transfusion-associated GVHD. Among the 73 reported cases, nearly all instances occurred in infants with recognized risk factors for which γ-irradiated cellular blood components already are recommended (ie, underlying congenital immunodeficiency disease, intrauterine and/or exchange transfusions, and transfusions from blood relatives). Notably, only six of the 73 infants (8%) with transfusion-associated GVHD did not fit readily into a recognized high-risk group. Three of the six infants were born prematurely with birthweights and gestational ages of 720 g and 25 weeks, 1528 g and 30 weeks, and 855 g and 25 weeks. Thus, nearly all infants with a known propensity to develop transfusion-associated GVHD already receive γ-irradiated cellular blood components per existing practices. The justification for a "blanket" policy to γ-irradiate all cellular blood components transfused to infants of all birthweights can be debated—at least, on a purely scientific basis.[7]

Considerations in Choosing Irradiated Components

Determining local policy on whether to transfuse γ-irradiated cellular blood components to neonates is based on three considerations: 1) conviction that there is a scientific indication to do so; 2) need to conform to an established standard of practice; and 3) ability to safely provide γ-irradiated blood components to all neonates who need them. Regarding the first consideration, scientific data are convincing that γ-irradiation of blood components to prevent GVHD is needed, with rare exception, only for neonates in the recognized high-risk groups of those with congenital cellular immunodeficiency diseases, those receiving intrauterine transfusions or neonatal exchange transfusions, and those receiving cellular blood components from blood relatives.

Regarding the second consideration, a questionnaire was sent in 1994 to institutional members of the American Association of Blood Banks involved in neonatal transfusions. Among 243 responding hospitals, 84% transfused some infants with γ-irradiated blood components; 55% provided γ-irradiated blood components for preterm infants with a birthweight ≤1.0 kg, and 35% did so for all infants <4 months of age, regardless of birthweight. Other, published recommendations[10] range from selectively transfusing γ-irradiated cellular components only to recognized high-risk infants to a blanket policy for all infants. Thus, there is no universally accepted "standard of practice" to which all must conform.

Regarding the third consideration, it is difficult to always identify neonates, early in life, who have severe congenital immunodeficiency diseases and who should receive γ-irradiated cellular blood components. To avoid the problem of overlooking neonates truly at risk of transfusion-associated GVHD, many centers provide γ-irradiated cellular blood components to all infants until they reach a predetermined age, generally, ≥1 year of age.

Unfortunately, this "blanket" approach by some institutions creates a standard of practice for others and forces practices that create new problems and risks. For example, many hospital blood banks do not have blood irradiators on site and must obtain γ-irradiated RBC units from outside blood suppliers. Because these units are not transfused immediately, they must be stored. Potassium leaks from the red cells into the extracellular fluid so that within a few days after γ-irradiation, the potassium concentration reaches a plateau level of approximately 70 mEq/L[11]—with a range of 55 to 100 mEq/L depending on the storage solution and the quantity of extracellular fluid. Although the dose of potassium infused with each small-volume RBC transfusion is small and does not require RBC washing,[12] the high potassium concentration in the primary unit can be quite dangerous for large-volume transfusions (eg, given during surgery), and fatalities have been reported.

Summary

In conclusion, although preterm infants are immunodeficient, transfusion-associated GVHD has been reported almost exclusively in infants from recognized high-risk groups—infants who must receive γ-irradiated cellular blood components.[7] Although the "blanket" transfusion of γ-irradiated cellular blood components to all infants is difficult to justify scientifically, legal and logistic factors strongly influence practice. Clearly, tertiary-care hospitals commonly γ-irradiate cellular blood components transfused to all newborn infants and continue this practice until the age at which severe immunodeficiency disorders become clinically evident. These disorders can be recognized by recurrent infections, diarrhea, failure to grow, distinctive morphologic and laboratory features (eg, great vessel anomalies and hypocalcemia in DiGeorge syndrome), lymphocytopenia, absence of lymphoid tissue, and a family history of other infants with similar problems—all of which become evident to a wary observer within the first several months of birth. Thus, it is reasonable to γ-irradiate cellular blood components for all infants at least until the age of 4 or 6 or 12 months—depending on the likelihood that immunodeficient infants will be managed at individual hospitals. However, one can debate the merit of "blanket" γ-irradiation for blood components transfused at community hospitals to otherwise healthy infants undergoing "routine" surgical and medical procedures.

Leukocyte-Reduced Components

The leukocytes in RBC and platelet units contribute to several undesirable complications of blood transfusions (Table 33), and the intent of removing the vast majority of WBCs from these components is to prevent their occurrence in patients at risk. Defining patients at risk is a matter of considerable controversy, with all physicians agreeing that most multitransfused hematology patients, oncology patients given intense chemotherapy, recipients of hematopoietic progenitor cell and solid organ allograft transplants, and premature neonates are at risk for these complications (Table 33) and should receive leukocyte-reduced blood components. However, some physicians believe that all transfused patients are at risk and, accordingly, favor universal leukocyte reduction of all cellular blood components transfused to all patients.[13] Scientifically, transfusion of leukocyte-reduced blood components to selected, at-risk patients is easily justified (Table 33). Those electing to practice universal leukocyte reduction must be

Table 33. Transfusion Complications Caused by WBCs

- Nonhemolytic transfusion reactions (commonly called "febrile nonhemolytic transfusion reactions")*
- Alloimmunization to HLA Class I antigens*
- Cytomegalovirus infections*
- Graft-vs-host disease†
- Immune modulation‡

*Efficacy of leukocyte reduction has been established for prevention.
†Leukocyte reduction is neither effective nor recommended.
‡Role of leukocyte reduction is controversial.

willing to accept the high cost and questionable medical benefit of this practice.[14]

Indications for Leukocyte-Reduced Components

The selection of leukocyte-reduced blood components for neonatal transfusions was reviewed several years ago,[15] and the conclusions were that leukocyte reduction could not be justified in the following instances: 1) to prevent nonhemolytic transfusion reactions because of their rarity in infants, 2) to prevent alloimmunization to HLA Class I antigens because it is an uncommon event and produces no known adverse effects during infancy, 3) to prevent GVHD because leukocyte reduction was ineffective when compared to γ-irradiation, or 4) to prevent immune modulation because its existence in transfused infants had not been established. However, it was clear that leukocyte reduction was a sound approach to prevent transfusion-transmitted CMV. Information reported since the previous review[15] supports the earlier conclusions—specifically, 1) nonhemolytic transfusion reactions continue to be reported only rarely during infancy,[16-18] 2) antibodies to WBC antigens have not led to clinically evident problems that require intervention,[15,19,20] 3) leukocyte reduction diminishes the risk of transfusion-transmitted CMV, 4) it is not recommended to prevent transfusion-associated GVHD, and 5) posttransfusion immune modulation has not been clearly demonstrated to produce clinically significant problems that require intervention by leukocyte reduction in infants.[15,21]

[Note added in proof: A recent report[22] suggested that prestorage leukocyte reduction of blood components transfused to preterm infants was associated with improvements in several clinical outcomes, but not with reductions in mortality or bacteremia. Unfortunately, as pointed out by the authors, the study was retrospective and had several potential limitations and biases. Thus, it does not provide definitive information.]

Summary

In conclusion, transfusing infants with leukocyte-reduced blood components can be justified on a sound scientific basis only to prevent transfusion-transmitted CMV. Sufficient data do not exist to warrant leukocyte reduction to prevent the other posttransfusion complications caused by leukocytes. Obviously, these complications will be possibly "ameliorated" serendipitously when leukocyte reduction is performed to prevent CMV, and controlled studies may never be conducted in infants to establish the efficacy of leukocyte reduction for each of the issues. As a final practical point, leukocyte reduction of blood components to be dispensed in small aliquots for neonatal transfusions is most easily and effectively accomplished at the time of collection (ie, prestorage).

Components that Are Negative for Sickle Hemoglobin

Individuals with sickle trait have red cells containing approximately 50% sickle hemoglobin (hemoglobin S) and 50% hemoglobin A; they are healthy and can donate units of blood with normal appearing red cells. Under most circumstances, RBC units from sickle trait donors are indistinguishable from normal units and can be transfused without complications to benefit patients requiring red cell replacement. However, under conditions of extreme hypoxia, acidosis, or both, patients with sickle trait can experience a sickle cell crisis. Theoretically, patients transfused with large quantities of sickle trait RBCs sufficient to convert them to an "acquired sickle trait" status could suffer a sickle cell crisis. Hence, the American Association of Blood Banks has recommended that transfusion services define patient populations who should be transfused with RBCs known to lack hemoglobin S.[23]

Knowledge both of the medical history of sickle trait patients and of the physiology of sickle hemoglobin and red cells with normal hemoglobin predicts that occasional patients converted to an acquired sickle trait status by relatively massive transfusion of sickle trait donor red cells will experience sickle crisis under conditions of hypoxia, acidosis, or both. However, definitive data are not available to accurately predict specific clinical or laboratory risk factors for this event. Accordingly, policies of various transfusion services may differ regarding which patients should be transfused with red cells known to lack hemoglobin S. Reasonable recommendations (Table 34) are based on one of two principles: either 1) only one or two RBC units will be transfused as the therapeutic dose (eg, infants) and, hence, must not be from sickle trait donors or 2) red cells containing sickle hemoglobin are already present in the recipient before transfusion so that transfusion of sickle trait red cells will diminish the effectiveness of treating sickle hemoglobin disorders by transfusions. In other massive transfusion settings involving patients without underlying sickle hemoglobinopathies (eg, cardiac bypass, liver trans-

---

Table 34. Patients for Whom Transfused RBC Units Should Be Hemoglobin S Negative

- Recipients of intrauterine and neonatal exchange transfusions
- Infants undergoing cardiac bypass or extracorporeal membrane oxygenation
- Preterm infants given repeated transfusions from the same RBC unit
- Patients who have sickle hemoglobin disorders and are undergoing erythrocytapheresis and simple or exchange transfusions

plantation, extensive surgery, erythrocytapheresis or exchange transfusion of nonsickle hemoglobin disorders) who are large enough to receive multiple RBC units, the testing of all RBC units before transfusion is difficult to justify because it is likely that only occasional or rare units will be from sickle trait donors. Thus, it is extremely unlikely that the posttransfusion quantity of sickle trait red cells in the recipient's bloodstream will be clinically significant.

References

1. Leukocyte reduction to prevent transfusion-transmitted cytomegalovirus. Association Bulletin No. 97-2. Bethesda, MD: American Association of Blood Banks, 1997.
2. Tegtmeier GE. The use of cytomegalovirus-screened blood in neonates. Transfusion 1988;28:201-3.
3. Preiksaitis JK, Brown L, McKenzie M. Transfusion-acquired cytomegalovirus infection in neonates: A prospective study. Transfusion 1988;28:205-9.
4. Strauss RG. Leukocyte-reduction to prevent transfusion-transmitted cytomegalovirus infections. Pediatr Transplant 1999;3:19-22.
5. Brady MT, Milam JD, Anderson DC, et al. Use of deglycerolized red blood cells to prevent posttransfusion infection with cytomegalovirus in neonates. J Infect Dis 1984; 150:334-9.
6. Bowden R, Sayers M. The risk of transmitting cytomegalovirus infection by fresh frozen plasma. Transfusion 1990;30:762-3.
7. Strauss RG. Data-driven blood banking practices for neonatal RBC transfusions. Transfusion 2000;40:1528-40.
8. Bowden RA, Slichter SJ, Sayers MH, et al. Use of leukocyte-depleted platelets and cytomegalovirus-seronegative red blood cells for prevention of primary cytomegalovirus infection after marrow transplant. Blood 1991;78:246-50.

9. Nichols WG, Price TH, Gooley T, et al. Transfusion-transmitted cytomegalovirus infection after receipt of leukoreduced blood products. Blood 2003;101:4195-200.
10. Hume HA, Preiksaitis JB. Transfusion associated graft-versus-host disease, cytomegalovirus infection and HLA alloimmunization in neonatal and pediatric patients. Transfus Sci 1999;21:73-95.
11. Jeter EK, Gadsden RH, Cate JC. Irradiation effect on aging red blood cells. Ann Clin Lab Sci 1991;21:420-5.
12. Strauss RG. Routinely washing irradiated red cells before transfusion seems unwarranted (invited commentary). Transfusion 1990;30:675-7.
13. Vamvakas EC, Blajchman MA. Universal leukocyte reduction: The case for and against. Transfusion 2001;41:691-712.
14. Dzik WH, Anderson JK, O'Neill SF, et al. A prospective, randomized clinical trial of universal WBC reduction. Transfusion 2002;42:1114-22.
15. Strauss RG. Selection of white cell-reduced blood components for transfusions during early infancy. Transfusion 1993;33:352-7.
16. Strauss RG, Burmeister LF, Johnson K, et al. AS-1 red blood cells for neonatal transfusions: A randomized trial assessing donor exposure and safety. Transfusion 1996;36:873-8.
17. Strauss RG, Burmeister LF, Johnson K, et al. Feasibility and safety of AS-3 red blood cells for neonatal transfusions. J Pediatr 2000;136:215-19.
18. Holman P, Blajchman MA, Heddle N. Noninfectious adverse effects of blood transfusion in the neonate. Transfus Med Rev 1995;9:277-87.
19. Strauss RG, Cordle DG, Quijana J, Goeken NE. Comparing alloimmunization in preterm infants after transfusion of fresh unmodified versus stored leukocyte-reduced red blood cells. J Pediatr Hematol Oncol 1999;21:224-30.
20. Bedford Russel AR, Rivers RP, Davey N. The development of anti-HLA-antibodies in multiply transfused preterm infants. Arch Dis Child 1993;68:49-51.

21. Wang-Rodriguez J, Fry E, Fiebig E, et al. Immune response to blood transfusion in very-low-birthweight infants. Transfusion 2000;40:25-34.
22. Ferguson D, Hébert PC, Lee SK, et al. Clinical outcomes following institution of universal leukoreduction of blood transfusions for premature infants. JAMA 2003;289:1950-6.
23. Fridey JL, ed. Standards for blood banks and transfusion services. 22nd ed. Bethesda, MD: American Association of Blood Banks, 2003:51.

INDEX

Page numbers in italics represent tabular material

A

ABO blood typing
    of children, 58, *73*
    in prenatal testing, 56
ABO compatibility
    and acute transfusion reactions, 114
    of blood components, 9, 10
    of Cryoprecipitated AHF, 31
    of granulocytes, *9*, 32, 33
    of hematopoietic transplants, 81, *82-83*, 84
    of plasma components, *9*, 23, 28
    of platelets, 20-21, *69*
ABO hemolytic disease of the newborn, 52, *53*, 55-56
Activated Factor VII, *101*, 104-105
Activated partial thromboplastin time (aPTT)
    and fresh frozen plasma use, 26, 27
    reference values of, 95, *96*
    in screening for coagulation disorders, 94
Acute extravascular hemolytic transfusion reaction (AEHTR), 126
Acute hemolytic transfusion reactions (AHTR), 114, *115-116*, 126-127. *See also* Transfusion reactions
Acute intravascular hemolytic transfusion reaction (AIHTR), 114, 126
Acute normovolemic hemodilution, 36
Additive solutions, 5, 12, 40
Administration of components
    Cryoprecipitated Antihemophilic Factor, 31
    Granulocytes, 35
    plasma components, 28
    Platelets, 22
    Red Blood Cells, 10, 12
    solutions in, 128
Adverse reactions. *See* Transfusion reactions
AEHTR (acute extravascular hemolytic transfusion reaction), 126
AHF. *See* Cryoprecipitated Antihemophilic Factor
AHTR (acute hemolytic transfusion reactions), 114, *115-116*, 126-127
AIHTR (acute intravascular hemolytic transfusion reaction acute), 114, 126
Air embolism, 65
Albumin, *3*, 28
Aliquots
    of fresh frozen plasma, 28-29
    of platelets, 22
    of red cells, 12
Allergic transfusion reactions, 130-131
    caused by FFP, 28
    management of, *118-119*
    washed RBCs for, 16, 131
Alloantibodies
    in HDF/HDN, 51-52, *53-54*, 55-56
    HLA, 38-39, 70, 132-133
    neutrophil, 70, 132-133
    platelet, 66-67, 77, 79-81
    selection of red cells with, 9-10
    in sickle cell patients, 74, 75
Alloimmune cytopenias
    and ABO-incompatible hematopoietic transplantation, 81-84
    alloimmune thrombocytopenia, 77, 79-81
    hemolytic disease of the fetus and newborn, 51-66
    neonatal alloimmune neutropenia, 70-71
    neonatal alloimmune thrombocytopenia, 66-69
    overview of, 51
    and sickle cell disease, 72-78

Alloimmune thrombocytopenia, 77, 79-81
Alloimmunization
  in HDF/HDN, 51-55
  to HLA antigens, 33-34, 38-39
  to neutrophil antigens, 70
  to platelet antigens, 66-67, 72
  in sickle cell disease, 72, 74-76
Alpha$_2$-antiplasmin, 105
Alpha$_2$-macroglobulin, 97, 105, 106
Aminocaproic acid, 80-81
Amniocentesis, 57, 58
Amniotic fluid analysis, 57
Amphotericin B, 33
Anaphylactic transfusion reactions, 16, 131
Anemia. *See also* Sickle cell disease
  dietary supplementation for, 17
  erythropoietin for, 17
  in preterm infants, 7-8
  Red Blood Cells for, 5
  symptoms in neonates, 6
Antibody screening
  in children, 10, 73
  in prenatal testing, 56
Antibody titers, 57
Anti-c, 51, 53, 55
Anticoagulant system, 105-108
  disorders of, 106-108
  in neonates, 105-106
Anticoagulant-preservative solutions, 1, 5, 13
Anti-D, 51-52, 53, 55, 57, 66
Antifibrinolytic therapy, 106
Anti-Fy^a (Duffy), 52, 53, 55
Antigen matching, 73, 76
Antigens
  HLA, 33-34, 38-39
  human neutrophil, 70, 132-133
  human platelet, 66-67, 77, 79-81
Anti-Jk^a (Kidd), 54, 55
Anti-K1 (Kell), 51-52, 53, 55, 57, 66
Antithrombin
  in anticoagulant system, 105
  concentrates, 106
  deficiency of, 106
  reference values for, 97

Apheresis platelets. *See* Platelets Pheresis
Apnea, 134
aPTT. *See* Activated partial thromboplastin time
Arrhythmias, 65, 135-136
AS solutions, 13
Autoantibodies, 74-75
Autologous Red Blood Cells, 36-38

B

Bacterial contamination
  of aliquots, 12-13
  transfusion reactions due to, 122, 133-134
  of umbilical cord blood, 38
Bacterial sepsis
  due to bacterial contamination, 133-134
  and exchange transfusions, 65
  and granulocyte transfusions, 32
  and T-activation, 127-128
Bilirubin
  in HDF/HDN, 54-55, 57, 64
  and hemolytic transfusion reactions, 129
Bilirubin encephalopathy, 54
Bleeding disorders
  Hemophilia A, 99, 102-103
  Hemophilia B, 99, 102, 103-104
  platelet dysfunction, 92-93
Bleeding times, 91-92, 96
Blood components
  bacterial contamination of, 12-13, 122, 133-134
  CMV-reduced, 149-153
  Cryoprecipitated Antihemophilic Factor, 3, 29-31
  granulocytes, 2, 31-35
  Hb S negative, 159-161
  irradiated, 15-16, 153-157
  leukocyte-reduced, 2, 3, 22, 157-159
  for patients undergoing ECMO, 39-40
  plasma components, 3, 23-29
  Platelets, 3, 17-22
  Red Blood Cells, 1, 2, 5-16

Red Blood Cells Washed, 2, 16-17, 131, 136
Blood loss, acute, 5
Blood warming, 128-129, 134
Bovine thrombin, 30-31

C

Calcium
   and exchange transfusions, 64-65
   and massive transfusion, *124,* 135
Cardiac arrest, 134
Cardiac arrhythmias, 65, 135-136
Cardiopulmonary bypass, 13-14, 36
CCI (corrected platelet count increment), 79, *80*
CD40 ligand, 130
Chagas' disease, 142-143
Chills, 129
Circulatory overload, 65, *120,* 131-132
Citrate toxicity, 64, 65
CJD (Creutzfeldt-Jakob disease), 143
Closure times, 92
CMV. *See* Cytomegalovirus
Coagulation factors
   concentrates of, 99, *100-101*
   in Cryoprecipitated AHF, 29
   deficiencies of
      coincident processes in, *98*
      contact factors, 94
      in hemophilia A, 99, 102-103
      in hemophilia B, 103-104
   in fresh frozen plasma, 23
   in neonates, 21
   in procoagulant system, 94
   reference values for, *96-97*
   replacement of, 95, 98, 99
   summary of, *24-25*
Coagulation tests, *96-97*
Colloidal solutions, 28
Component therapy. *See also* Blood components
   after ABO-incompatible hematopoietic transplantation, 81, *82-83,* 84
   concept of, 1
   for ECMO patients, 39-40

Corrected platelet count increment (CCI), 79, *80*
CPDA, *13*
Creutzfeldt-Jakob disease (CJD), 143
Cryopoor plasma, 27
Cryoprecipitated Antihemophilic Factor (AHF)
   administration of, 31
   and CMV, 152
   contraindications and precautions for, 31
   description of, *3,* 29
   dosage of, 31
   indications for, *3,* 29-31, 99
   transfusion volumes for, *11*
   use in ECMO, 40
Cryosupernatant, 27
Crystalloids, 28
Cytokines, 114, 130
Cytomegalovirus (CMV), 149-153
   clinical significance of, 151-152
   and granulocyte transfusions, 33
   and leukocyte reduction, 15, 158-159
   patients at risk for, 150-151
   prevention of, 152-153
   seronegative components, *70,* 152-153
Cytopenia. *See* Alloimmune cytopenias

D

D antigen
   in HDF/HDN, 51-52, 59-60
   in platelet transfusions, 21
   in red cell transfusions, 9
   weak, 59-60
DAT. *See* Direct antiglobulin test
DDAVP, 93, 102
Dedicated units, 12-13
Deglycerolized Red Blood Cells, 151
DEHP (di-2-ethylhexyl phthalate), 139
Delayed hemolytic transfusion reactions (DHTRs), 74, 137. *See also* Transfusion reactions
Desferoxamine, 77, 138-139
Dexamethasone, 32

DIC (disseminated intravascular coagulation), 27, 107
Di-2-ethylhexyl phthalate (DEHP), 139
Dilutional coagulopathy, 65
Direct antiglobulin test (DAT), 20, 58
Directed donations, 38-39
Disseminated intravascular coagulation (DIC), 27, 107
Donor-specific units
    autologous red cells, 36-38
    directed donations, 38-39
Doppler ultrasound, 57, 58
2,3-DPG (2,3-diphosphoglycerate), 13-14
Duffy blood group
    in delayed hemolytic reactions, 137
    in HDF/HDN, 51-52, *53*

E

ECMO
    age of RBCs in, 13-14
    component therapy in, 39-40
Embolism, air, 65
Encephalopathy, bilirubin, 54
Epstein-Barr virus, 142
Erythropoietin, 17, 65-66
Exchange transfusion
    age of RBCs in, 13-14
    and hypocalcemia, 135
    in sickle cell disease, 76-77, *78*
    in treatment of HDF/HDN, 61, *62-63*, 64-65

F

Factor II (prothrombin), *96*
Factor IX
    concentrates, *101, 102,* 103-104
    deficiency of, 99, 103-104
    reference ranges for, *97*
Factor V, 23, 28, *97*
Factor V mutation, 107, 108
Factor VII, *97*
Factor VIIa concentrates, *101,* 104-105
Factor VIII
    concentrates, 93-94, *100,* 102-103
    in Cryoprecipitated AHF, 29
    deficiency of, 31, 99, 102-103
    in plasma components, 23, 28
    reference ranges for, *97*
Factor X, *97*
Factor XIII, 29
Febrile nonhemolytic transfusion reactions (FNHTR), 15, *117,* 129-130
Fetal blood sampling, 57-58, 68
Fetomaternal hemorrhage (FMH), 55, 60-61
Fever, *117,* 129-130
FFP. *See* Fresh Frozen Plasma
Fibrin sealants, 30
Fibrinogen
    in Cryoprecipitated AHF, 29, 31
    quantitative assay for, 94
    reference values for, *96*
Fibrinolytic proteins, 95, *97*
Fibrinolytic system, 105-108
    disorders of, 106-108
    in neonates, 105-106
Filtration
    for Cryoprecipitated AHF, 31
    for Granulocytes, 34
    for leukocyte reduction, 14-15
    for plasma components, 28
    for RBCs, 11-12
FMH (fetomaternal hemorrhage), 55, 60-61
FNHTR (febrile nonhemolytic transfusion reactions), 15, *117,* 129-130
Folate deficiency, 17
Fresh Frozen Plasma (FFP)
    administration of, 28
    aliquots of, 28-29
    and CMV, 152
    contraindications and precautions for, 27-28
    description of, *3,* 23
    dose of, 23, 27, 28
    and hypocalcemia, 135
    indications for, *3,* 23, 27, 99
    jumbo plasma, 23, 28-29
    transfusion volumes for, *11*

use after ABO-incompatible hematopoietic transplantation, *82-83*
use in ECMO, 40

G

Gamma irradiation. *See* Irradiation
G-CSF (granulocyte colony-stimulating factor), 31-32, 71
Glucose, blood, *125,* 134, 136
Glucose-6-phosphate dehydrogenase (G6PD), 129
Graft-vs-host disease. *See* Transfusion-associated graft-vs-host disease
Granulocyte colony-stimulating factor (G-CSF), 31-32, 71
Granulocytes Pheresis
    ABO compatibility of, *9,* 32, 33
    administration of, 35
    contraindications and precautions for, 33-34
    description of, *2,* 31-32
    dosage of, 35
    indications for, *2,* 32-33, 71
    transfusion volumes for, *11*

H

HBV (hepatitis B virus), *140,* 141
HCV (hepatitis C virus), 140-141
HDF/HDN. *See* Hemolytic disease of the fetus/newborn
Hemapheresis, therapeutic, 81
Hematocrit, of Red Blood Cells, 5
Hematopoietic transplantation
    and directed donations, 38-39
    transfusion support following ABO-incompatible, 81, *82-83,* 84
Hemoglobin
    in neonates, 5-6
    in preterm infants, 7-8
Hemoglobin S negative components, 129, 159-161
Hemoglobinopathies
    sickle cell disease, 8, 72-*78*
    thalassemia, 8

Hemoglobinuria, 129
Hemolysis. *See also* Hemolytic disease of the fetus/newborn
    and blood warming, 128-129, 134
    drug-induced, 127
    nonimmune, *117,* 128-129
Hemolytic disease of the fetus/newborn (HDF/HDN)
    blood group systems involved in, *53-54*
    clinical features of, 55-56
    laboratory diagnosis of, 56-58
    pathogenesis of, 51-55
    prevention of, 58-61
    selection of red cells for, *62-63*
    treatment of, 61, 64-66
Hemolytic transfusion reaction syndrome, 74
Hemolytic transfusion reactions (HTRs)
    acute, 114, *115-116,* 126-127
    delayed, 74, 137
    and sickle cell disease, 74-77, *78*
Hemolytic-uremic syndrome (HUS), 20, 27
Hemophilia A
    calculating dosages for, 102-103
    description of, 99, 102
    treatment of, 29, 102-103, 104-105
Hemophilia B
    calculating dosages for, *102,* 103-104
    description of, 103-104
    treatment of, 99, 104-105
Hemorrhage
    fetomaternal, 55, 60-61
    intracranial, 67
    intraventricular, 95
    periventricular, 95
Hemosiderosis, 138-139
Hemostasis
    anticoagulant and fibrinolytic systems in, 105-106
    overview of, 91
    platelet function in, 91-93
    procoagulant system in, 94-95, 98
    screening tests for, 94

Heparin-induced thrombocytopenia (HIT), 20
Hepatitis, 140-141
HIV (human immunodeficiency virus), *140,* 141
HLA alloimmunization
    and directed donations, 38-39
    and granulocyte transfusions, 33-34
    and leukocyte reduction, 15, 158
    and neutropenia, 70
    and TRALI, 132-133
HPA. *See* Human platelet antigens
HTLV-I/II (human T-cell lymphotropic viruses), *140,* 142
HTR. *See* Hemolytic transfusion reactions
Human immunodeficiency virus (HIV), *140,* 141
Human neutrophil antigens (HNA), 70
Human platelet antigens (HPA), 66-67, 77, 79-81
Human T-cell lymphotropic viruses (HTLV-I/II), *140,* 142
Humate-P, 93, 99
HUS (hemolytic-uremic syndrome), 20, 27
Hydrops fetalis, 54
Hyperbilirubinemia
    in HDF/HDN, 54-55, 58, 64
    and hemolytic transfusion reactions, 129
Hyperglycemia, 136
Hyperhemolysis, 74
Hyperkalemia
    in exchange transfusion, 65
    and irradiation, 15-16, 135
    management of, *123*
    and nonimmune hemolysis, 129
Hypersplenism, 20
Hypervolemia, 65, *120,* 131-132
Hypocalcemia
    in exchange transfusion, 64-65
    management of, *124*
    in massive transfusion, 135
Hypoglycemia, *125,* 134, 136
Hypothermia, *122,* 134

I

ICH (intracranial hemorrhage), 67
Identification of patient, 114
Idiopathic thrombocytopenic purpura (ITP), 20, 67, 68
IgA deficiency, 16, 131
Immunomodulation, 15, 154
Infants, preterm
    defined, 1
    hemorrhagic disease in, 27
    periventricular hemorrhage in, 95
    platelet transfusions in, 18-20
    procoagulant proteins in, 95, *96-97*
    Red Blood Cells for, 7-8
    safety of additives for, 12
    serial transfusions in, 12-13
    use of FFP in, 27-28
Infections, posttransfusion
    Creutzfeldt-Jakob disease, 143
    cytomegalovirus, 149-153
    and directed donations, 38
    due to bacterial contamination, *122,* 133-134
    Epstein-Barr virus, 142
    and exchange transfusions, 65
    hepatitis, 140-141
    HIV, 141
    HTLV, 142
    parasitic infections, 142-143
    parvovirus B19, 142
    variant Creutzfeldt-Jakob disease, 143
    West Nile virus, 142
Infectious disease testing, 35
Inhibitor proteins, 95, *97*
Intracranial hemorrhage (ICH), 67
Intrauterine transfusions, 61, *62-63,* 65
Intravenous immunoglobulin (IVIG)
    for treatment of alloimmune thrombocytopenia, 80-81
    for treatment of NAIT, 68, 69
Intraventricular hemorrhage (IVH), 95
Iron chelation therapy, 77, 138-139
Iron deficiency anemia, 17

Iron overload, 77, 138-139
Irradiation, 15-16, 153-157
    of granulocytes, 34
    and hyperkalemia, 15-16, 135
    patients who should receive
        components, *154*
    of platelets, *69*
    to prevent TA-GVHD, 15, 34,
        138, 153-157
ITP (idiopathic thrombocytopenic purpura), 20
IVH (intraventricular hemorrhage), 95
IVIG. *See* Intravenous immunoglobulin

J

Jaundice, 64
Jumbo plasma, 23, 28-29

K

Kell blood group, 51-52, *53*
Kernicterus, 54-55
Kidd blood group
    in delayed hemolytic reactions, 137
    in HDF/HDN, *54,* 55

L

Lead exposure, 139
Leukocyte reduction
    benefits/disadvantages of, 15
    and CMV, 150-153, 158-159
    of directed donations, 39
    and febrile nonhemolytic transfusion reactions, 129-130, 158
    indications for, 157-159
    methods of, 14-15
    and TRALI, 133
    and variant Creutzfeldt-Jakob disease, 143
Leukocyte-reduced Platelets, *3,* 22
Leukocyte-reduced Red Blood Cells, 2

M

Malaria, 142
Massive transfusion
    age of RBCs in, 13-14
    and hyperkalemia, 135
    hypocalcemia in, *122,* 135
Mechanical hemolysis, *117,* 128
Microaggregate filters, 11

N

NAIT. *See* Neonatal alloimmune thrombocytopenia
NAN. *See* Neonatal alloimmune neutropenia
Necrotizing enterocolitis (NEC), 65, 127-128
Neonatal alloimmune neutropenia (NAN)
    clinical features of, 70-71
    laboratory diagnosis of, 71
    pathogenesis of, 70
    treatment of, 71
Neonatal alloimmune thrombocytopenia (NAIT)
    clinical features of, 67
    laboratory diagnosis of, 68
    pathogenesis of, 66-67
    treatment of, 68-69
Neonates. *See also* Preterm infants
    ABO group of, 10
    alloimmune neutropenia in, 70-71
    alloimmune thrombocytopenia in, 66-69
    antibody screen in, 10
    anticoagulant and fibrinolytic system in, 105-106
    coagulation proteins in, 27, 95
    Cryoprecipitated AHF for, 31
    dedicated units for, 12-13
    directed donations for, 39
    hemolytic disease of the newborn, 55-66
    hemolytic transfusion reactions in, 126-127
    hemorrhage in, 27, 95
    irradiated components for, 155-157
    platelet function in, 91-92
    platelet transfusions in, *19*
    pretransfusion testing in, *73*

procoagulant proteins in, 95, *96-97,* 98
Red Blood Cells for, 5-7, 10
transfusion volumes for, 10, *11*
use of filters for, 11-12
Neutropenia
and granulocyte transfusions, 32-33
neonatal alloimmune, 70-71
Neutrophils
antigens/antibodies, 70, 132-133
normal counts in infants, 71
Nonimmune hemolysis, *117,* 128-129
Nucleic acid amplification testing (NAT), 141
Nutritional support, 28

P

PAI (plasminogen activator inhibitor), 105
Parasitic infections, 142-143
Partial thromboplastin time (PTT)
and fresh frozen plasma use, 26, 27
reference values of, 95, *96*
in screening for coagulation disorders, 94
Parvovirus B19, 142
Patient identification, 114
Percutaneous umbilical blood sampling, 57
Perioperative blood recovery, 36, 37
Periventricular hemorrhage, 95
Phototherapy, 61, 65
Plasma components
ABO compatibility of, *9,* 23, 28
administration of, 28
aliquots of, 28-29
and allergic reactions, 131
contraindications and precautions for, 27
cryosupernatant, 27
description of, *3,* 23
dose of, 28
indications for, *3,* 23, 26-27
jumbo plasma, 23, 28-29
and T-activation, 128
thawed plasma, 23, 28
Plasma frozen within 24 hours, 23

Plasmin, 105
Plasminogen, *97*
Plasminogen activator, 105
Plasminogen activator inhibitor (PAI), 105
Plasticizer exposure, 139
Platelet aggregation studies, 92
Platelet concentrates
ABO/Rh compatibility of, 20-21, *69*
administration of, 22
bacterial contamination of, 133, 134
calculating dose of, 21-22
CMV reduced risk, *69*
contraindications and precautions of, 20-21
description of, *3,* 17-18
indications for, *3,* 18-20
irradiated, *70*
leukocyte-reduced, *3,* 22
pooled, 17-18
refractoriness to, 72, 79
transfusion volumes for, *11*
in treatment of NAIT, 68-*69*
used after ABO-incompatible hematopoietic transplantation, *82-83*
volume reduction of, 21, 22, 132
Platelets. *See also* Platelet concentrates; Platelets Pheresis; Thrombocytopenia
antigens/antibodies, 66-67, 77, 79-81
dysfunction of, 18, 29-30, 92-93
function in neonates, 91-92
normal counts of, *96*
refractoriness to, 72, 79
response to transfusions, 79
Platelets Leukocytes Reduced, *3,* 22
Platelets Pheresis (PP)
ABO compatibility of, 20-21
aliquots of, 22
calculating dose of, 21-22
contraindications and precautions of, 20-21
description of, *3,* 18

indications for, *3*, 18-20
leukocytes reduced, *3*, 22
PLTs. *See* Platelets
Pooled components
    Cryoprecipitated AHF, 31
    platelets, 17-18
Posttransfusion purpura (PTP), 81
Potassium
    in exchange transfusion, 65
    and irradiation, 15-16, 135
    management of, *123*
    and nonimmune hemolysis, 129
Prenatal testing, 56
Preoperative autologous donation, 36, 37
Preterm infants
    defined, 1
    hemorrhagic disease in, 27
    periventricular hemorrhage in, 95
    platelet transfusions in, 18-20
    procoagulant proteins in, 95, *96-97*
    Red Blood Cells for, 7-8
    safety of additives for, 12
    serial transfusions in, 12-13
    use of FFP in, 27-28
Pretransfusion testing, *73*
Procoagulant system, 94
    abnormalities of, 98-99, 102-105
    in neonates, 95, 98
    reference values for, *96-97*
Protein C, *97*, 105, 107
Protein S, *97*, 105
Prothrombin G20210A mutation, 107-108
Prothrombin time (PT)
    and fresh frozen plasma use, 26, 27
    reference values for, 95, *96*
    in screening for coagulation disorders, 94
PT. *See* Prothrombin time
PTP (posttransfusion purpura), 81
PTT. *See* Partial thromboplastin time
Purpura fulminans, 107

R

Recombinant antithrombin concentrate, 106
Recombinant Factor IX, 103
Recombinant Factor VIII, *100*, 102
Red Blood Cells Leukocytes Reduced, *2*, 14-15
Red Blood Cells Washed, *2*, 16-17, 131, 136
Red Blood Cells
    ABO/Rh compatibility of, *9*
    aliquots of, 12, 132
    autologous, 36-38
    changes in storage of, 13-14
    composition of, 1, *2*, 5
    description of, 1, 5
    filters for, 11-12
    frozen, 151
    indications for, *2*, 5-8
    irradiation of, 15-16, 153-157
    leukocyte-reduced, *2*, 14-15, 157-159
    modification of, 14-16
    for neonates, 5-7, 10
    for patients older than 4 months, *6*, 9
    for premature infants, 7-8
    selection of, 8-12, *62-63*
    for sickle cell disease, 8
    special considerations for, 12-16
    for thalassemia, 8
    transfusion volumes for, *11*
    use in ECMO, 40
    use in HDF/HDN, *62-63*
    washed, *2*, 16-17, 131, 136
Rh blood group
    in HDF/HDN, 51-52, *53*
    in platelet selection, 21
    in red cell selection, 9
    testing, 56, 58, *73*
Rh Immune Globulin (RhIG)
    composition and indications for, *4*
    in prevention of HDF/HDN, 52, 58-61
    use in platelet transfusions, 21
Rigors, 129, 130
Rituximab, 81

S

Sepsis
    due to bacterial contamination, 133-134
    and exchange transfusions, 65
    and granulocyte transfusions, 32
    and T-activation, 127-128
Sickle cell disease (SCD)
    pretransfusion testing in, *73*
    red cell alloimmunization in, 72, 74-77
    red cell transfusions in, 8
    simple vs exchange transfusion in, 76-77, *78*
Single-donor platelets. *See* Platelets Pheresis
Solutions
    additives, 5, 12, 40
    anticoagulant-preservatives, 1, 5, *13*
    colloids, 28
    in component administration, 128
Storage of RBCs, 13-14
Stroke, 77

T

T lymphocytes, 154
T-activation of red cells, 127-128
TA-GVHD. *See* Transfusion-associated graft-vs-host disease
Thalassemia, 8
Thawed plasma, 23, 28
Thrombin, 30-31, 105
Thrombin time (TT), 94
Thrombocytopenia
    alloimmune, 77, 79-81
    and exchange transfusions, 65
    heparin-induced, 20
    idiopathic thrombocytopenic purpura, 20
    neonatal alloimmune, 66-69
    platelets for, 18
    in posttransfusion purpura, 81
Thrombophilia, 107
Thrombosis
    in antithrombin deficiency, 106
    and Factor V mutation, 107, 108
    in Protein C deficiency, 107
    and prothrombin G20210A mutation, 108
Thrombotic thrombocytopenic purpura/hemolytic-uremic syndrome (TTP/HUS), 20, 27
TRALI (transfusion-related acute lung injury), *121,* 132-133
Transfusion reactions
    acute, 113-136
    allergic/anaphlyactic, *118-119,* 130-131
    bacterial contamination, *122,* 133-134
    caused by WBCs, *158*
    circulatory overload, *120,* 131-132
    Creutzfeldt-Jakob disease, 143
    cytomegalovirus infection, 149-153
    delayed, 136-143
    Epstein-Barr virus, 142
    of exchange transfusion, 64-65
    febrile nonhemolytic, 15, *117,* 129-130
    from granulocyte transfusions, 33, 35
    hemolytic, 114, *115-116,* 126-127, 137
    hemosiderosis, 138-139
    hepatitis, 140-141
    HIV, 141
    HTLV, 142
    management of, *115-125*
    metabolic complications, *123-125,* 134-136
    nonimmune hemolysis, *117,* 128-129
    parasitic infections, 142-143
    parvovirus B19, 142
    plasticizer and lead exposure, 139
    posttransfusion purpura, 81
    procedures for, 113-114
    sickle cell transfusion reaction syndrome, 74

T-activation of red blood cells, 127-128
thermal effects, *122,* 134
transfusion-associated graft-vs-host disease, 137-138
transfusion-related acute lung injury, *121,* 132-133
variant Creutzfeldt-Jakob disease, 143
West Nile virus, 142
Transfusion-associated graft-vs-host disease (TA-GVHD), 137-138
   choosing irradiated components for, 155-156
   and directed donations, 38
   and irradiation, 15, 34, 138, 153-157
   patients at risk for, 153-155
Transfusion-related acute lung injury (TRALI), *121,* 132-133
Transfusions
   ABO compatibility of, 9, 10
   after ABO-incompatible hematopoietic transplantation, 81, *82-83,* 84
   in children less than 4 months, 5-8, 10, 12-13, 18-20
   in children more than 4 months, 6, 9-10, *19*
   of Cryoprecipitated AHF, *11,* 29-31
   exchange, 135
      in sickle cell disease, 76-77, *78*
      in treatment of HDF/HDN, 61, *62-63,* 64-65
   filters for, 11-12
   of granulocytes, *11,* 32-35
   intrauterine, 61, *62-63*
   massive, *122,* 135
   of plasma components, *11,* 23, 26-29
   of Platelets, *11,* 18-22, 68-*69*
   rate of administration, 10, 12
   of Red Blood Cells, 5-12
   serial, dedicated units for, 12-13
   in sickle cell disease, 75-77, *78*
   in treatment of HDF/HDN, 61, *62-63,* 64-65
   volumes for, 10, *11*
Transfusion-transmitted diseases, 140-143
   Creutzfeldt-Jakob disease, 143
   cytomegalovirus, 149-153
   Epstein-Barr virus, 142
   hepatitis, 140-141
   HIV, 141
   HTLV, 142
   parasitic infections, 142-143
   parvovirus B19, 142
   variant Creutzfeldt-Jakob disease, 143
   West Nile virus, 142
Transplantation. *See* Hematopoietic transplantation
Trypanosoma cruzi, 142-143
T4:T8 ratio, 154
TTP/HUS (thrombotic thrombocytopenic purpura/hemolytic-uremic syndrome), 20, 27

U-V

Umbilical cord blood, 36, 38
Variant Creutzfeldt-Jakob disease (vCJD), 143
Viral infections, posttransfusion
   cytomegalovirus, 149-153
   Epstein-Barr virus, 142
   and exchange transfusions, 65
   hepatitis, 140-141
   HIV, 141
   HTLV, 142
   parvovirus B19, 142
   viral window-period risk of, *140*
   West Nile virus, 142
Vitamin K, 27
Volume expansion, 27-28
Volume overload, 65, *120,* 131-132
Volume reduction of components, 21, 22, 132
Von Willebrand disease, 29, 31, 92-94
Von Willebrand Factor (vWF)
   in neonates, 92

reference ranges for, *96*
replacement of, 99, 101

W

Warfarin, 26-27
Warming blood, 128-129, 134
Washed Red Blood Cells
    for allergic transfusion reactions, 16, 131
    description of, *2*, 16
    and hyperkalemia, 136
    indications for, *2*, 16
Weak D antigen, 59-60
West Nile virus (WNV), 142
Whole Blood, 36
    ABO compatibility of, *9*
    composition of, *4*
    and hypocalcemia, 135
    indications for, *4*, 36